To my daughters,
Sophie, Emma, Sasha

CONTENTS

Illustrations

Acknowledgments

This book has been in the making for a long time. Initial ethnographic fieldwork was conducted as part of a research project on religious conversion, carried out while I was based at the Max Planck Institute for Social Anthropology between 2003 and 2006. But it was only after I took up a position at the London School of Economics and Political Science that the project expanded and slowly morphed into a book about the dynamics of conviction, and for which I conducted additional ethnographic fieldwork in the period between 2008 and 2013.

I am heavily indebted and very grateful to those who accompanied me on parts of the fieldwork. Himia Suerkulova was my United Nations Volunteers (UNV) counterpart back in 1998 and 1999, and assisted me for a month in 2004 while conducting a series of interviews with specialists and officials; Damira Umetbaeva was an excellent research assistant from 2003 to 2004 when she was still an undergraduate, and has since then become a close friend and colleague; Nurgul introduced me to the spiritual world of clairvoyants and healers, a world that otherwise would have remained largely invisible to me; Emil Nasritdinov collaborated with me in a related research project on former mining towns, and invited me to travel with the Tablighi Jamaat on several of its mission trips. Particular gratitude goes out to Kadyr Osmonov, who, together with his wife, Aziza, was an excellent host and became a close friend. It was with great sadness that I learned of his untimely death in 2011.

I have benefited from the institutional funding of the Max Planck Institute for Social Anthropology, and am grateful to its director, Chris Hann, for pointing out some of the larger theoretical implications of what was then still a modest project. Most of the writing was conducted during a one-year sabbatical at the LSE. Sections of two chapters have appeared in previous publications. Portions of chapter 4 were published in a much shorter publication titled "Awkward Secularity between Atheism and New Religiosity in Post-Soviet Kyrgyzstan," in the volume *Atheist Secularism and Its Discontents: A Comparative Study of Religion and Communism in Eurasia*, edited by T. Ngo and N. Quijada (2015). Parts of chapter 6 appeared in "Mediating Miracle Truth: Permanent Struggle and Fragile Conviction in Kyrgyzstan," in *The Anthropology of Global Pentecostalism and Evangelicalism*, edited by S. Coleman and R. Hackett (2015).

Early chapter drafts were presented at workshops and departmental seminars: in the UK at Brunel University, SOAS, the University of Kent, University of Oxford, Sussex University, and the University of East London; in Central Asia at the L.N. Gumilyov Eurasian National University and the American University of Central Asia; and in Germany at the Humboldt University, the Max Planck Institute for Cultural Diversity, and the Max Planck Institute for Social Anthropology. Special thanks to Julie McBrien, Deniz Kandiyoti, Julie Archambault, David Pratten, Emil Nasritdinov, Damira Umetbaeva, Isak Niehaus, David Henig, Narmala Halstead, Marloes Janson, Jon Mitchell, Svetlana Jacquesson, Philipp Schröder, Yuliya Shapoval, and Manja Stephan-Emmrich for asking pertinent questions and for offering the possibility to present ideas that were often still embarrassingly underdeveloped. It was a privilege to present three of the book's chapters at my home department's Friday Seminar and to receive the thoughtful and critical feedback of my colleagues, including Matthew Engelke, David Graeber, Fennella Cannell, Michael Scott, Alpa Shah, Deborah James, Katy Gardner, Harry Walker, Hans Steinmuller, Stephan Feuchtwang, Maurice Bloch, Laura Bear, Catherine Allerton, Rita

Astuti, Charles Stafford, Nick Long, and Gisa Weszkalnys. The detailed comments of the two anonymous reviewers were invaluable for making this book a stronger one, as was the editorial guidance of Roger Malcolm Haydon and Jim Lance at Cornell University Press. I am especially thankful to Bruce Grant, for his critical, thoughtful, and detailed comments on the penultimate draft of this book. Finally, my greatest gratitude goes to my partner, Judith Bovensiepen, for her teasing critiques, demands for clarity, and loving support, which not only enabled the completion of this book, but made the writing process so much more enjoyable than it otherwise would have been.

A Note on Transliteration
and Translation

In transliterating Russian from the Cyrillic I have used the Library of Congress system. For Kyrgyz I have used the same system with the exception of the following letters: ө = ö and ү = ü. When appropriate I have placed the original terms in parentheses, indicating whether they are Kyrgyz or Russian terms. I have not done this in all instances because several key words are used in both languages and because many of the spiritual and political terms are linked less to a "national" language than to a religious or political tradition. All translations are my own, except where noted.

FRAGILE CONVICTION

INTRODUCTION

Ideational Power in Times of Turmoil

As we marched through the streets, I felt full of energy. It was scary when the riot police attacked us, but we managed to push back. Somehow I felt strong, and then stronger still when other groups joined us. There was a lot of cheering. I was like, Wow, I never knew that so many people were against [President] Akaev.... At the time I was convinced [*uveren*] that what we were doing was important. For me it was about democracy and freedom, and about fighting against corruption. I was convinced that if we succeeded, things would be better.... When I came home [to the shared flat] that afternoon, I found the other girls sleeping. I was amazed that they were not even aware of what was going on. [Later] they were critical of my involvement because they knew that my parents were against me being involved. But I was just amazed that they didn't care.... At that point I did not have doubts. My first doubt, as you call it, happened the day after the revolution [when shops were being looted]. We formed patrols to protect the shop owners; it was dangerous. Aigerim, who had joined [the youth movement] KelKel[1] at the same time as me, mentioned to me, "This looting was not supposed to happen." That is when I started to doubt. Also because the atmosphere [in KelKel] had changed; it became clear that many [of its members] had joined for their own interests. For me it had been about discussing ideas and the future of our country.... Maybe I was also trying to fill a void in myself; to be part of a group like this felt good. But for many of the others it was about something else, about supporting a family member or about pushing their own careers. We had these meetings [in the weeks after the Tulip Revolution].
The discussions were no longer about ideas. It was all about dividing up the trips [abroad], about who would speak where.... I got fed up with it, and left. Later on I started to read about the problems with democracy [as a concept] and about NGOs and how they were financed from the West. And I was disappointed in [the new president] Bakiev. My KelKel acquaintances from back then would say, "Yes, Bakiev is terrible, but still it is good that the revolution happened." Personally I don't know if it was good or bad.

Mirgul's account² of her experiences with the youth movement KelKel and her involvement in the Tulip Revolution of April 2005 provides a brief reflection on a situation that was at first hopefully embraced as a means to the peaceful displacement of a corrupt government, but ultimately resulted in widespread disillusionment when the prevailing opposition leader, Kurmanbek Bakiev, instated a regime that was even more objectionable than that of his predecessor, Askar Akaev.³ The intensity of the event, as much as its ephemeral and ultimately disillusioning qualities, is reflective of Kyrgyzstan's tumultuous post-Soviet political trajectory, a period in which political and religious movements and prophets thrived, usually only for brief moments.

Situated in this turbulent environment, Mirgul's story directs attention to the mechanisms by which individuals become committed to a cause and gain certainty about the meaning and value of the ideas involved. For several weeks Mirgul had been convinced that the removal of President Akaev from office would result in more freedom and allow for a more democratic form of government, both of which were sacrosanct values to her at the time. Initially uncertain about the prospects for success, she was both surprised and emboldened by the realization that she and her fellow revolutionaries were supported in this struggle by a mass of people. In those moments she felt great clarity: the goals seemed clear and near, and motivation peaked. However, her certainty, commitment, and clarity turned out to be fleeting. When we first spoke about her experiences, three years after the revolution, she saw herself as having been terribly naive—still an undergraduate student—a young woman who had found herself caught up in the moment.

In this book I examine ideational power by focusing on the energy and momentum that are built into "flashes of conviction" like the one described by Mirgul. The focus is on the affective dimension of collective ideas, on the energy that both animates and exceeds societal structures.⁴ I analyze how ideas gain momentum when shared by a group of like-minded compatriots and the transformative potential these ideas can have when directed toward a clear goal or distinct enemy.

The brightness of the flash of conviction should, however, be examined in view of the flickering that came before and the afterglow left in its wake. That is, because conviction unfolds in real time, it needs to be looked at in relation to the doubts and hesitations that may precede or accompany it, and the satisfactions or disillusionments that may succeed such a flash. Mirgul's conviction was not diminished by her friends' criticism or her parents' disapproval. On the contrary, her sense of righteousness was intensified by their critique, just as the experience of warding off a police attack emboldened her. In fact, Mirgul's belief in and commitment to the cause eroded only after an *insider* (a friend and fellow KelKel member) started to express criticism. This set in motion a series of nagging doubts that were fed by the egotistic attitude of other KelKel members and the disappointing conduct of the new government. In this process, the signifiers "freedom" and "democracy" changed meaning, now referring to careerism and disagreeable geopolitical agendas. These shifts and changes demonstrate the importance of paying due attention to the social, epistemic, and affective dimensions of the making and unmaking of temporary conviction.

By using the concept of conviction I aim to draw attention to the fluctuating intensity and quality of attitudes, motivations, and beliefs. So how does this instance of momentary political clarity compare to other forms of conviction? I could equally have started this introduction with some of the other flashes of conviction that feature prominently in this book. For example, the account of a miracle at a Pentecostal church in southern Kyrgyzstan would have illustrated the affective energies released by collective prayer. A description of the application of rhythmic sound and touch by spiritual healers would have made the bodily sensations experienced by patients palpable. A sketch of the "inspired fellowship" (Turner 2012, back cover) among Tablighi Muslims during their proselytizing trips would have provided insight into how fantastical images become experienced as real. An account of the arrival of international aid workers in a destitute mining town would have illuminated the vital connections between hope, conviction, and disillusionment.

These instances of conviction have varying intensities, rhythms, and scopes, the documentation and comparison of which will serve to bring to light the various dimensions of ideational power. But the point is also that the described pattern—the swelling of momentum, the flash of intensity, the release of energy—points at a dynamic that exceeds the particularities of each instance of conviction. Referring to this dynamic as "pulsation," I theorize how ideational power is produced and released, and with what effects. Pulsation describes the trajectories of collective ideas whose intensity waxes and wanes over time. Moreover, as a sensitizing concept, pulsation indexes different aspects of ideational power: the assertion of ideas (the impulse), their traction within social fields (pressure), and their rhythmical patterns (throbbing). By taking this approach I aim to understand how people become convinced, and how they cease being convinced, of concrete assertions of truth. By analyzing different examples of conviction with a focus on the impulses and resonances generated by these assertions of truth, I will explain the strengths and weaknesses of collective ideas.

These topics are explored in the context of post-Soviet Kyrgyzstan at a time of economic collapse and political turmoil. The unsettling effects of "post-Soviet chaos" (Nazpary 2002) were felt with particular intensity in the mining town of Kokjangak, where most of the fieldwork for this book took place. Located in Jalalabad Province in southern Kyrgyzstan, it had largely been built between 1930 and 1950. Kokjangak had been a paragon of Soviet modernization, a frontier town[5] in a largely agricultural and underdeveloped region, its inhabitants depicted in official discourse as pioneers in the establishment of a new civilization. This formerly vibrant town had fallen hard after the collapse of the Soviet Union. Half of the population emigrated, many of its buildings were dismantled, and the remaining ten thousand residents tried to make a living through informal mining, limited agricultural activities, and circular migration. Kokjangak had come to resemble what Anna Tsing conceptualizes as chaos—"a frontier spun out of control, its proliferations no longer productive for the authorities" (2005, 43).

In these destitute conditions, new visions and ideas were actively asserted and hopefully embraced. Right after the Soviet collapse, neoshamanic practices boomed, and even two decades later there was still an impressive network of spiritual healers and visionaries in the town. From the mid-1990s onward, a range of development organizations initiated projects in Kokjangak, but despite being enthusiastically welcomed, they often produced more disappointment than satisfaction. In the early 2000s the Pentecostal Church of Jesus Christ set up a congregation that attracted a significant following. Not much later Deobandi-inspired versions of Islam gained ground, especially among the male youth. And in 2005 there was real excitement in the weeks before, during, and after the Tulip Revolution, especially because the opposition leader (and later president) Kurmanbek Bakiev had previously lived and worked in Kokjangak and might thus direct funds toward the town (a hope that never materialized). While new political and religious movements proved attractive in this context of economic hardship and social fragmentation, their failure to fulfill their own promises meant that "conversions" were often temporary. By documenting and describing how people in Kokjangak specifically and Kyrgyzstan more generally encountered and engaged with a range of charismatic and millenarian movements, in this book I offer an ethnographic tribute to the post-Soviet condition of uncertainty in Central Asia.

It could be objected that the theoretical focus on *fragile* instances of conviction, based on research in an *unstable* social field, presents an atypical case that has little value apart from being an exotic curiosity. But this would be missing the point. Rather, the "extreme" features of this study throw into high relief processes that have much wider resonance. In a world where power is "no longer routed so centrally through the state" (Ferguson 2004, 394), and which is characterized not only by transnational flows but also by isolation and disconnect, the workings of ideology are changing as well. There is something suggestive about Arjun Appadurai's argument that we are shifting from a "vertebrate" world of nation-states to a "nonvertebrate" or "cellular" world in which global flows rely on the infinite reproducibility of minimal ideological and functional principles (2006). If anything, this shift has made ideological processes less predictable and more volatile.[6] As I have argued elsewhere, precisely because nationalisms, populisms, and fundamentalisms have become so conspicuously present over the past two decades, "it is essential not to take their strength for granted, but to examine the dynamics of conviction and doubt through which their efficacy and affective qualities are made and unmade" (Pelkmans 2013, 1). That is, the focus on the making and unmaking of conviction in a context where the state-system has come undone and its ideological framework imploded provides a valuable vantage point from which to gain deeper insight into the workings of ideology in the contemporary world more generally.

In this book, the key question is how systems of ideas become animated, that is, how they come to matter in the lives of people. The concept "ideology" refers to such systems of ideas and forms the larger conceptual backbone of the book, but this is approached through "conviction," a useful lens for studying how ideologies are animated. "Conviction" is used to draw attention to the affective dimensions of belief, knowledge, and attitude, and suggests variation among subjects and fluctuations over time. "Ideology" foregrounds the issue of power, and thereby opens up possibilities for a political-economic analysis of ideation. Let me outline in more detail how

I employ these two contested concepts in order to lay the foundations for the conceptual framework that I develop in this book.

Ideology: Ideas and Power

The concept of ideology is a slippery one that has frustrated generations of scholars. A central problem is that because ultimately *all* ideas are bound up with power, the term is often considered too general to have analytical purchase. The problem can be detected even in the work of those who employ a concrete and straightforward definition of the term. Eric Wolf, for example, defines ideology as "unified schemes or configurations [of ideas] developed to underwrite or manifest power" (1999). When Wolf then applies the term to the cases in his book *Envisioning Power*, it becomes clear that he uses "ideology" at times to refer to "unified schemes" or doctrines that are actively propagated by elites, while at other times he employs it much more loosely to refer to ordered "configurations" of collective customs, practices, and ideas that indirectly "underwrite" the order of society. This is no critique of Wolf's work but rather an observation about the different ways in which ideas and power can be woven together. After all, dominant ideas not only are advanced through explicit doctrine, but they have a material existence in state institutions or rituals, and unwittingly filter our perceptions of reality. However, the result is that "the term ideology threatens to expand to vanishing point" (Eagleton [1991] 2007).[7]

Intriguingly, while these reflections may suggest that ideology is too pervasive to be analytically useful, a contrasting view suggests that we are living in a post-ideological era. This "end-of-ideology" position was first voiced over half a century ago, when scholars in the United States (e.g., Bell 1960) declared that "ideological distinctions" had become "devoid of social and psychological significance for most people" and that the existing abstract political ideologies "lack motivational potency and behavioral significance" (Jost 2006, 651). More recently, and more relevantly to the geopolitical context of this book, it was the erosion and then collapse of Soviet socialism that inspired ideas of the end of ideology, even "the end of history" in the sense that with the victory of capitalism there would be no longer any credible alternative ideologies left (Fukuyama 1989). Such end-of-ideology visions dovetailed with the frequently offhand depiction of the post-Soviet era as constituting an "ideological vacuum" (Buckley 1997; Karagiannis 2009, 93). This perceived vacuum was seen as problematic and dangerous precisely because it seemed to indicate the absence of collective values, which also translated into ideas of a "spiritual vacuum" (Vorontsova and Filatov 1994) and a "moral vacuum" (Wanner 2011, 214).[8]

Announcements of the death of ideology have always been rather contradictory, possibly because a vacuum easily becomes a site of turbulence, or, as Clifford Geertz put it, "It is a loss of orientation that most directly gives rise to ideological activity" (1973, 219). Not entirely surprising then is Terry Eagleton's exclamation that "it is announced that the concept of ideology is now obsolete," when in fact we are witnessing a "remarkable resurgence of ideological movements," as he wrote in response to Francis Fukuyama's claim about the death of ideology ([1991] 2007, xx).[9] Writing about ideological activity in Russia during the 1990s, Eliot Borenstein aptly commented that the post-Soviet condition is more appropriately described as one of ideological excess than ideological void, and provided "fertile ground for fantasies of an apocalypse" (1999, 439, 447). But this ideological excess, which refers to the conspicuous presence of nationalist, market, developmental, and religious visions, also suggests the fragility of each single ideology and the lack of a stable and dominant ideological framework.

What are we to do with these opposing stances concerning the ideology concept and the contradictory views about the role of ideology in the contemporary world? To clarify the discussion it is useful to momentarily adopt Slavoj Žižek's distinction between three modes of ideological operation: ideology in-itself, ideology for-itself, and ideology reflected into itself. The first, ideology in-itself, is the most explicit incarnation of ideology, which refers to the active assertion of "a doctrine, a composite of ideas, beliefs, concepts and so on, destined to convince us of its 'truth'" (Žižek 1994, 10). Second and somewhat more indirect are the "institutions, rituals and practices" that give "body" to ideology, rather similar to what Althusser ([1971] 2008) refers to as "ideological state apparatus" and includes all institutions (such as schools, museums, courts, regulatory bodies, etc.) that play a role in reproducing state ideology, whether directly or indirectly. Finally, ideology as "reflected into itself" refers to the "quasi-'spontaneous' presuppositions and attitudes" of self-declared non-ideological practices (Žižek 1994, 15). This ideological mode of operation is more or less what Bourdieu refers to as doxa, as that which "goes without saying because it comes without saying" (1977, 167–69). The point of bringing up these distinctions is to suggest, not only that those who speak about the absence of ideology and those who speak about its omnipresence might actually be talking about different modes of ideological power, but also that the relative weight of these different modes depends on the nature of society and the position of the relevant collective ideas within it.

In stable and well-integrated political systems the dominant ideas tend to be internalized and naturalized, making ideological work less conspicuous. For example, Žižek argues that in late capitalism the weight of "ideology as such is diminished: individuals do not act as they do primarily on account of their beliefs or ideological convictions—that is to say, the system . . . bypasses ideology in its reproduction and relies on economic coercion, legal and state regulations, and so on." But although "ideology has moved to the background [it] has by no means disappeared" (1994, 14–15). Rather, precisely because the dominant ideas have become part and parcel of people's common sense, they can be reproduced almost invisibly through the ideological state apparatus. Thus, what Daniel Bell (1960) and Fukuyama (1989) referred to as the "end-of-ideology" could also be seen as the epitome of ideological efficiency, of the temporary *hegemony* of a specific set of ideas within a particular sociopolitical configuration. In such a situation "dominant power" does not need to rally a population behind a greater cause or convince people to defend "the truth," but instead can rely on their pragmatic acquiescence.[10] The flipside of this is that the more ideology is naturalized—the more it comes to be taken for granted—the less it is able to directly motivate the sentiments and actions of people. Therefore, despite all the problems of Bell's end-of-ideology thesis, there is value in his implicit suggestion that there are situations in which ideologies no longer act as sets of belief capable of being "infused with passion" (1960).

By contrast, in situations of sociopolitical fragmentation and rapid societal change "ideology" moves to the foreground. This means that existing ideologies become denaturalized, first because in unstable situations the dominance of dominant power cannot be taken for granted, and second because ideology-infused common sense is challenged by changing circumstances. This may easily lead to the explicit defense as well as radicalization of dominant ideas.[11] Post-Soviet Central Asian corollaries are easy to point out. A good example of the intensification of dominant ideas would be the Stalin-style cult of personality that developed in Turkmenistan in the 1990s, in which the country's first president appeared as a latter-day Islamic prophet leading his chosen nation (see Hann and Pelkmans 2009). Different but equally conspicuous is the futuristic redesigning of Kazakhstan's capital, Astana, sometimes described as the "Dubai of the steppe," a glorification of ideas of modernity that are firmly rooted in the Soviet project (Buchli 2007; Laszczkowski 2011).

Similar state-directed tendencies toward "extreme expression" have been present in Kyrgyzstan, but none obtained semihegemonic status. Instead, the ideological landscape became more radically fragmented and was therefore frequently depicted as an "ideological vacuum," which, as we have seen, is simultaneously the terrain of ideology par excellence. That is to say, Kyrgyzstan essentially developed into a laboratory for testing out ideologies. Indeed, it was seen as a frontier and "mission field" by evangelicals, pious Muslims, and (secular) development specialists. Precisely because none of the advanced visions could rely on a stable ideological (state) apparatus, they became at once more conspicuous and volatile. The most disturbing example of this in Kyrgyzstan's recent history is the 2010 conflict, when ideas of ethnic purity, feeding on political and economic tensions, radicalized with such speed that towns and cities across the south of the country erupted in massive violence, resulting in hundreds of casualties (see chapter 1). In other words, when power fields are unstable, ideology becomes denaturalized, but this fragility of ideology simultaneously triggers its reassertion resulting in an ideological excess. From this perspective, Kyrgyzstan is a particularly interesting case in which to observe the workings of conviction in a "post-ideological" world and to draw attention to conviction's fragility.

Conviction: Power of Ideas

The concept of ideology is usually associated with *dominant* power,[12] but dominance is not what makes ideas powerful in the sense of potent or effervescent. In fact, there appears to be a partially inverse relationship between the "strength" (or tenacity) of ideology and its "potency" (as the ability to move people to action). This tension needs to be kept in mind when focusing on conviction. The "energized state" that I am trying to capture has been explored by many others, through the perspectives of charisma, collective effervescence, *communitas*, and affect. In their own specific ways, each of these terms tries to capture the emotive "energy" that is produced in the connections between individuals (such as leaders and followers), within liminal groups (made up of equals), and between humans and their environment. In this book I will make use of the insights generated through these approaches while applying them to the relationship between subjects and collective ideas.

There are several reasons why I propose *conviction* as the conceptual focus for a study of ideational power instead of using the more common alternatives. The first is that conviction connects the fields of religion and politics better than related terms such as "belief" or "opinion." Second, more so than opinion, disposition, attitude, and knowledge, the term "conviction" makes the affective dimension of the relationship between subject and ideas palpable. It is for this reason that I avoid the term in the plural, because to speak of people's religious or political convictions would be a labeling exercise characteristic of "topographic approaches" instead of an approach that is able to capture "processes" (Crapanzano 2004, 8). It is in the singular that the affective dimension comes to the fore, as conveyed when we refer to someone as being "full of conviction," another one as "lacking conviction," and a preacher (or politician or car salesman) as "speaking with conviction," that is, with clarity and purpose. The goal of this book is to understand how this quality of conviction is gained and lost, and to which actions or inactions this may lead.

In exploring the connections between people and collective ideas, Althusser's theory of interpellation ([1971] 2008) is a useful point of reference. His famous example, or "theoretical scene," of interpellation is that of a police officer who hails (interpellates) a person in the street by calling out "Hey, you," on which the person recognizes being addressed and turns around. In the moment of turning, that is, in the submissive response to the voice of ideology, the person is (re)produced as a subject through a process of mutual recognition. Althusser depicts interpellation as an internal process in which individuals "are *always-already* subjects" (46, italics in the original); that is, he presents ideological interpellation as an unfailing mechanism in the production of subjects. This suggests, quite clearly, that Althusser works with a concept of society in which different tenets of ideology form a coherent whole that is durably integrated with the socioeconomic fabric of that society.[13] Unfortunately, this seamless depiction of interpellation is unhelpful for understanding of ideational power in fragmented ideological landscapes, where the ideological state apparatus has collapsed and/or where new ideologies assert themselves. The question, therefore, is how can we make productive use of the idea of interpellation (without necessarily clinging to the term itself) and apply it to fragmented ideological landscapes?

I argue that the three elements of interpellation—the voice of ideology, the response of the listener, and the mutual recognition—need to stay at the center of analysis, while rejecting the assumptions that permeate Althusser's writing. Whereas for Althusser the "voice of ideology" is quintessentially that of the state, we need to look at concrete and nonhegemonic assertions of religious, political, and economic truths. While Althusser seems to assume that the listener's response is conditioned by guilt and a concomitant desire for the law,[14] this needs to be complemented with attention to the more immediate needs and desires that make subjects reach out to certain instantiations of ideology and ignore or reject others. And while for Althusser the outcome of interpellation is one of blanket submission, we need to ponder possibilities such as ideological ambivalence and rejection (by "bad subjects") or enthusiastic embrace (by neophytes, for example), and study its variation within a population, as well as how this changes over time.

I use the concept of pulsation for exactly this purpose: to explore the instability of the links between these elements without presuming the effect of the configuration and moreover to draw attention to the generative capacity of ideology as opposed to assuming a finalized result. Pulsation is first of all about the *impulse* or the voice of ideology: the proclamations of a future of abundance through the neoliberal gospel; of health and prosperity for those who accept Jesus in their hearts; of peace and happiness for those who follow the ways of the Prophet. This also makes one wonder about the kind of impulses that were generated by assertions of "scientific atheism," and how this may be related to the difficulties in producing devoted atheists (see chapter 3). As Thomas Csordas has argued (2007, 261), some messages are better transposable and certain practices more portable, something that has immediate relevance for the ability to bind and invigorate new and old subjects.

This bring us to the second aspect of pulsation, namely that the impulse needs to trigger a meaningful response. I argue that the voice of ideology can gain traction only when there is a productive tension. Whether we take Marx's view that the articulation of protest starts with the "sigh of the oppressed creature" ([1844] 2002, 171) or follow Foucault's argument that "where there is desire, the power relation is already present" (1978, 81), for the voice of ideology to be heard there needs to be a gap between a desired horizon and a detested reality. The Tablighis and Pentecostals promised to release people from the bonds of slavery caused by addiction and illness; the development specialists proclaimed that they would end poverty; the revolutionary leaders that they would bring an end to corruption. Moreover, the voice of ideology can only produce commitment and conviction for as long as its utopian horizon is seen as realistic and in reach.[15]

Finally, pulsation refers to the rhythmic fluctuation (or resonance) that the mutual recognition may produce. This can be seen as a form of Emile Durkheim's collective effervescence, in which people's "very act of congregating [generates] a sort of electricity [that] launches them to an extraordinary height of exaltation" (1915, 217–18). Or, to use Victor Turner's term *communitas*, it is among equals who temporarily come together in situations of liminality that we find the highest levels of commitment and conviction (1969). While acknowledging the value of these older works, in this book I emphasize that the buildup and release of such affective energies is a precarious affair plagued by contradictions. Throughout the book, I explore the ideological fervor generated among church congregations, religious travel groups, and revolutionaries. Similar to Durkheim's collective effervescence and Turner's *communitas*, these intense experiences of togetherness tended to be limited in duration, as were the clarity of vision, the commitment to a goal, and the conviction of truth that accompanied the experiences.

Pulsation triggers many questions, including about what kinds of collective ideas are attractive under what conditions, and about how communal bonds may generate conviction. As has been pointed out above, not only do ideological voices assert themselves most explicitly and forcefully in contexts of fragmentation and crisis, it is also then that mutual recognition is particularly fragile. All this makes a comparative analysis of different ideological "voices" in such contexts particularly worthwhile.

The Book

It is now more than twenty years ago that I first ended up in Kyrgyzstan. At the time of my first visit I was an undergraduate student in anthropology who spent his summers traveling through Eastern Europe. One of those was the summer of 1994, when a friend and I hitchhiked from Amsterdam to Warsaw, took a train to Moscow, and there, although lacking the necessary visas, bought tickets for a train that took us through Kazakhstan to Kyrgyzstan's capital, Bishkek, where we arrived seventy-two hours later.[16] Kyrgyzstan had been independent for merely three years and was going through a deep economic crisis. People were struggling, nostalgic about the past, but also hopeful about the future.

Intrigued by the people I met and the challenges they faced, I decided to return the following year to carry out five months of fieldwork for my master's thesis, which I did in the provincial city of Karakol in northeastern Kyrgyzstan. Back then I was primarily interested in people's adjustments to, and interpretations of, the new market economy. This specialization landed me a job with the United Nations Development Programme (UNDP) in 1998, when I was tasked with setting up a poverty alleviation program in Jalalabad Province (*oblast'*). It was during this one-year stay that I also began to work in Kokjangak, the mining town that later would become my primary field site.

When I realized that international development was not my calling, I decided not to renew my contract and moved away from Central Asia to conduct my PhD research in the Georgian border region with Turkey. Chance had it that in 2003 I returned to Kyrgyzstan to study missionary encounters and dynamics of religious conversion, as part of a Max Planck Institute for Social Anthropology research program on religion and civil society. Much of the research data presented in this book was collected during this fourteen-month fieldwork period. However, the materials for several topics (chapter 3 on atheism and chapter 4 on Tablighi Islam) were collected during shorter research visits (totaling six months) between 2008 and 2013. In fact, it was only during those later years that my earlier interests in (political and economic) uncertainty and my subsequent interests in (religious) beliefs and practices came together in a project on conviction, that is, in a project that connects the anthropology of politics and of religion.

I recount my personal trajectory because it has contributed significantly to the shape of this book. The relatively long duration of research has allowed me to relate the events and encounters that form the empirical core of most chapters to the slower-paced shifts and changes of Kyrgyzstan's ideological landscape (see especially chapter 1). My long-term involvement has also made it possible to make an informed selection of ethnographic cases to illuminate complementary aspects of the dynamics of conviction.

It would have been possible to present this book as a contribution to the study of religion, given the attention to changes in the religious landscape throughout, and the inclusion of two chapters about concrete religious movements—the Tablighi Jamaat in chapter 4 and a Pentecostal church in chapter 5. However, such a framing would push the chapter that focuses on neoliberalism and nationalism (chapter 1) to the margins, and leave those on atheism (chapter 3) and spiritual healing (chapter 6) hanging in an uncomfortable position. But the issue has ramifications beyond those of textual organization. The point is, as Maurice Bloch has argued, that "no valid theoretical distinction can be made between the transcendental social and the 'religious'" (2013, ix). Setting it apart from what he calls the "transactional social," the transcendental, for Bloch, refers to those aspects of life that draw on the imagination, whether we tend to categorize these as social, political, or religious (Bloch 2008, 2060). And that is ultimately what this book is about: documenting the ways in which people orient themselves to transcendental values and utopian horizons, following the trajectories of collective imaginations in uncertain conditions, observing how existential, epistemological, and ontological concerns merge in the struggle for a livable future.

This, then, brings us back to Mirgul's story of the Tulip Revolution with which this introduction began. The story highlighted the role of the transcendental in political struggle and emphasized that conviction is ultimately about the epistemic, emotive, and social processes that propel the connection with a utopian horizon. When Mirgul reached out to the ideas of democracy and freedom, she did so by identifying with a group of like-minded others who attempted to realize a common goal. This utopian horizon receded, indeed revealed itself as a ploy for careerist and geopolitical interests, as soon as the revolution was won and the group of revolutionaries disbanded. The ideas of democracy and freedom turned out to be moving targets—"floating signifiers"—with increasingly disillusioning qualities. As such, this story was also about the volatile context, one in which political and religious movements emerged and receded, in which hope and disillusionment quickly followed each other. It is to this topic that I now turn.

Part I

Uncertain Times and Places

1

Shattered Transition

The Reordering of Kyrgyz Society

Located in the middle of Bishkek, Kyrgyzstan's capital, Ala-Too Square stands out for its immensity and emptiness. Created in 1984 to mark the sixtieth anniversary of the Kyrgyz Soviet Socialist Republic (SSR), it was designed to accommodate oversized state spectacles and military parades. The square is traversed by two parallel roads and lined with buildings covered in marble: a massive cube that houses the National History Museum to the north; the presidential office building, or White House, behind a row of poplars in the northwest; arched white buildings along the square's east and west flanks; and, to the south, the robust Ministry of Agriculture, behind which the snow-covered Ala-Too Mountains can be seen on clear, smog-free days.

If a time-lapse video had been made of the square between 1984 and the present day, it would reveal meaningful details about the political rhythms and their transformations in Kyrgyzstan over those three decades. During the first seven years of coverage, the video would draw attention to the yearly Victory Day celebrations and October Revolution parades that punctuated time in what was then a quiet, Soviet provincial backwater. Those expecting to see turbulence in the period directly before or after Kyrgyzstan gained independence, on August 31, 1991, would be disappointed—the square remained eerily quiet, a visual indicator of the reticence and wariness with which the political elite and the population at large greeted the disintegration of the Union of Soviet Socialist Republics.[1] The economic crisis of the 1990s caused the square to deteriorate, leaving the fountains waterless and causing the pavement to crack open, which even the colorful new state spectacles such as those on Independence Day could not conceal. It was not until the turn of the century that the square began to play a more active role in the public life of the newly independent country. Collective prayers started to fill the square at the end of Ramadan (*orozo ait*) and the Feast of the Sacrifice (*kurban ait*), marking the return of Islam to public life and triggering debate about the proper place of religion in an ostensibly secular state. In this period the square also became an important site for expressing political discontent, featuring frequent demonstrations and meetings, and forming the center stage of two revolutions. During the largely peaceful Tulip Revolution of March 2005, the square was occupied by students and others dressed in pink and yellow shirts, before groups of young men stormed and occupied the White House (Lewis 2008, 142). Similarly, in April 2010 the square filled up just before the grand finale, when demonstrations culminated in an open clash with security forces, resulting in a battle in which at least eighty-six people lost their lives and numerous buildings around the square were burned down.

These public events are suggestive of the rhythms of Kyrgyz political life, and the issues that fueled collective action. We will return to these events, but not before considering the more slow-paced ideological currents that informed them. To gain an overview of these slower trends we could do worse than to take our time-lapse video camera and zoom in on the three statues that successively occupied the square's central fifteen-meter-high pedestal. In 1984, the first statue to adorn what was then still named the Lenin Square was, unsurprisingly, a statue of Lenin, ten meters tall and with his outstretched right arm pointing southward toward the Ala-Too mountain range. What is unique about this Lenin is that he remained standing on his pedestal long after 1991. While in the following months and years Lenins were being removed from the central squares of most Soviet successor state capitals, Bishkek's Lenin ended up

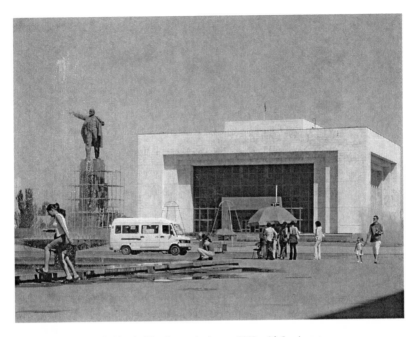

Bishkek's Ala-Too Square in August 2003, with Lenin statue,
soon to be removed, and the National History Museum

having a longer post-Soviet than Soviet life by the time he was moved in 2003. Then, at midday on August 16, Lenin was carefully lifted from his pedestal, watched in silent protest by only a handful of people waving a flag of the USSR.[2] But instead of being destroyed, Lenin was reinstalled only a hundred meters away behind the National History Museum, placed on a lower pedestal, faced northward, with his outstretched hand pointing to the *Jogorku Kenesh* (parliament) and the American University of Central Asia.

Back on Ala-Too Square, the statue replacing Lenin was the *Erkindik* (Liberty) statue, modeled after the Greek goddess of liberty but given a Kyrgyz face and holding in her outstretched hand not a torch but a *tunduk*, the wooden centerpiece of the roof of a yurt and symbol of the Kyrgyz nation. It might be fitting that Erkindik oversaw two revolutions (in 2005 and 2010), but this was a "liberty" quite different from what Akaev, Kyrgyzstan's first president, had envisioned when he commissioned the statue. Erkindik had been designed to underscore the values of democracy and sovereignty that Akaev's government had promoted since independence, and which had earned the country the international reputation as an "island of democracy" in the mid-1990s. However, as soon as Erkindik was placed on her pedestal, she started to draw criticism, ranging from objections to her short-sleeved dress that revealed too much bare bronzed skin and was therefore deemed non-Kyrgyz and un-Islamic, to the complaint that holding the *tunduk* is a sacrosanct act reserved for elderly men, and suspicion that the president's wife had been the model for Erkindik's face (see Cummings 2013, 612–13).

Plans to replace Erkindik were made under the authoritarian presidency of Kurmanbek Bakiev, who had come to power after the Tulip Revolution of 2005 and was ousted in Kyrgyzstan's second revolution, in 2010. Bakiev had consulted with advisers and artists about the construction of a new statue, but "most of the concepts put forward were too local or marginal, and thus unsustainable and unworkable at a national level" (Morozova 2008, 19). As a result, Erkindik remained on the square until 2011, when she was unceremoniously removed and replaced by the solid national hero Manas, who was seated in full armor on his mighty stallion.

Manas was a legendary medieval king who had united the forty Kyrgyz tribes to lead them to victory on the battlefield, as narrated in the *Epic of Manas*. This epic poem developed over centuries, and although several versions have been written down since the late nineteenth century, it continues to be recited orally by narrators called *manaschi*. Since independence, the epic and its hero have become a key symbol of the nation-building effort, increasingly presented as the epitome of Kyrgyz culture (van der Heide 2008). Despite official attempts to boost Manas's internationalist credentials, this Kyrgyz symbol was ultimately exclusionary for many of the republic's non-Kyrgyz citizens (see also Wachtel 2013, 977). The Manas statue, designed by a Kyrgyz sculptor and cast in bronze in Moscow, was said to have arrived in Kyrgyzstan in 2011 on *Kadyr-tun* (the holy night of the Ramadan) and was unveiled during *Orozo ait*, cleverly tapping into a combination of religious and nationalist sentiment that had become increasingly prominent during the preceding years.

The passing away of the communist Lenin, who made way for the liberal Erkindik, who in turn was replaced by the national hero Manas, provides one glimpse of the ideological shifts that unfolded in Kyrgyzstan. But while the succession of statues reflects broader ideological currents, it

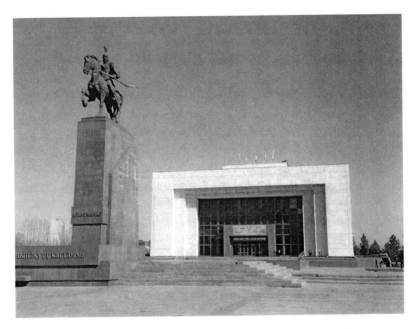

Bishkek's Ala-Too Square with the new Manas statue, April 2014

does so in a rather out-of-sync manner. Thus, Lenin entered the square at a moment when the Soviet Union was already in decline, and he outlived the USSR by more than a decade. Likewise, Erkindik was erected in 2003 when the "freedom" buzz of the 1990s had lost its allure and "democratic" president Akaev had become increasingly autocratic, only two years before he was ousted in the Tulip Revolution. Finally, although the medieval Manas with his message of Kyrgyzness was supposed to be timeless, he entered the square after Kyrgyz nationalism had shown its dark side during clashes with the Uzbek minority in June 2010, and after the new government had pledged to promote an inclusive model of statehood.[3]

Statues, and certainly statues on the central squares of capital cities, carry significant symbolic weight. They are designed to root state ideology in territory (literally anchoring it to the soil), to make abstract ideas concrete (even give them a face), and to allow otherwise fleeting messages to transcend time (by making them immemorial). These are some of the reasons why the toppling of prominent statues—Saddam Hussein in Baghdad, Lenin in Kiev—are powerful symbolic gestures that mark the end of epochs, bold acts that desacralize former leaders or ideologies (Verdery 1999; Grant 2001). Similarly, the erection of a new statue can be a powerful act of inaugurating a new beginning or marking a passage. Clearly these potentials informed the rotation of statues on Ala-Too Square; they were erected and removed to signal ideological change and to legitimate state power. However, the delays in the removal of Lenin and then Erkindik, and the belatedness, whether in arrival or departure, of all three statues, illustrate the difficulties that successive regimes experienced in gaining and maintaining symbolic hegemony. If we agree with Philip Abrams (1988) that the "nature of state power lay first and foremost in its ideational force, as a discursive effect of political discourse" (Grant 2001, 336; see also Comaroff and Comaroff 2000, 322–23), then the awkward dance of statues on Ala-Too Square revealed the difficulty of producing a "state idea" able to infuse a sufficiently sacred aura, one providing the legitimacy and authority necessary for effective government. Indeed, Lenin's belated removal and the ridiculing of Erkindik, as well as Erkindik's and Manas's untimely arrivals, highlighted the precariousness of producing symbols sufficiently encompassing and powerful to connect with the population at large and instill a sense of inclusion and purpose.[4]

So what was being symbolized? I already noted that the succession of socialist, liberalist, and nationalist statues reflected real changes in the larger ideological landscape, even if the timing was off. But there is more to it. Lenin's gaze projected a communist utopia onto the Kyrgyz horizon, his arm gesturing the people toward this bright future. By contrast, Erkindik's message of liberty failed to outline a future, relying instead on the universal trope of "freedom" that was as detached from the local reality as she herself was floating through the air. And Manas—well, he stands firmly on the ground, but his gaze is primarily directed into a mythical past determined by kinship relations. The succession of statues, then, suggests the gradual loss of political vision, the erosion of progressive civic ideology. Moreover, while Lenin reached out to all nations, such an encompassing stance remained unrealized by his successors. Erkindik mixed Kyrgyz particularity with a universal vision of freedom but did so unsuccessfully, while the archetypal Kyrgyz hero Manas represented an ethnic world with which few Russians, Uzbeks, or representatives of other minorities identified. The statues seem to have become not only increasingly shortsighted but also exclusionary, changes that, as we will see, have had real-time parallels in Kyrgyzstan's recent political history.

Obviously none of the above claims, which are based on a reading of just three statues, should be taken at face value. Instead they should be seen as hypotheses to be examined by following the trajectories of socialism, (neo) liberalism, and nationalism in the post-Soviet period. In the remainder of this chapter I explore how these ideologies translated into political practice, and analyze the tensions between rhetoric and reality that has characterized Kyrgyzstan's so-called transition. Moreover, by connecting the succession of statues to the political events unfolding on the square and beyond we can see how Kyrgyzstan's unraveling transition became interspersed with recurrent eruptions of political turmoil. This complex relationship provides insight into the reconfigurations of political and social space in the decades that followed the Soviet collapse.

Projections of Transition

"Transition" has the dubious honor of being one of the terms used most frequently to characterize post-Soviet trajectories, both by those who lived through the period and by those who observed and wrote about it. Although the dictionary meaning of "transition" is simply a period of change from one to another relatively stable situation, in its application to postsocialist countries, "transition" obtained distinct teleological qualities, that is, the observed changes were all viewed in relation to a predetermined final endpoint. As others have noted, transition ideas were essentially a slightly modified version of modernization theory, both of which convey a linear progressive and teleological kind of thinking, assuming the final stage to be a version of market democracy (e.g., Carothers 2002).

These assumptions drove the reform agenda of the first independent government of Kyrgyzstan headed by President Askar Akaev. In the early 1990s, when the country was on the brink of economic collapse, Akaev's government opted for a transition strategy of "shock therapy" and closely cooperated with the International Monetary Fund (IMF), the World Bank, and various multilateral development institutions to carry out a comprehensive structural adjustment program. The reforms included the liberalization of markets, the privatization of property, and the reduction of welfare programs. Kyrgyzstan introduced its own currency in May 1993, and by mid-1997 it had privatized approximately two-thirds of the state sector (Anderson 1999, 71). Preparations for this comprehensive restructuring of the economy were carried out in close cooperation with international organizations. To illustrate, over 50 percent of bills passed through parliament in the 1990s were drafted by international organizations and international NGOs (Cooley and Ron 2002, 19). No surprise then that Kyrgyzstan became essentially the poster child for the Washington consensus. For example, a high-ranking Western diplomat commented in 1994 that "politically, Kyrgyzstan is light-years ahead of the other new republics. Economically, it is carefully and methodically preparing the way for a market economy."[5]

Although international pressure on Kyrgyzstan's government to adopt the structural adjustment package was significant, it would be wrong to see the Akaev government as merely a passive recipient of an externally imposed neoliberal agenda. In fact the president was a very vocal spokesperson of (neo) liberal ideology (Anderson 1999, 81). Possibly his rather excessive references to former US presidents such as Abraham Lincoln and Thomas Jefferson (Akaev 1993, 9, 18; see also McGlinchey 2011, 87; Cummings 2013) were intended to impress US donors, but they were also indicative of the kind of future society he envisioned. A good example is a published speech from 1993 in which Akaev presented a straightforward view of the direction of transition. He started by positing that Kyrgyzstan would have been prosperous if not for "some irrational path in history" due to which the country spent "seventy years . . . in the grip of a totalitarian system" (1993, 10–11). The way to rectify this perceived historical travesty was full-out liberalization: religious freedom, political freedom, economic freedom (1993, 11–12). This was neoliberalism in almost its purest form, which optimistically hoped (or naively assumed) that when given "freedom," society would rid itself of the imposed "irrationalities" and be guided by a natural or intrinsic drive toward the final destination of liberal modernity.

The labels by which Kyrgyzstan came to be known, such as the "Switzerland of Central Asia" and "island of Democracy," referred not just to the economic sphere but also to the promotion of "freedom of information, a free press, and freedom of association" (Akaev 1993, 22), which had resulted in a significantly more pluralistic media landscape than existed in neighboring countries, and the emergence of a range of nongovernmental organizations. Attracted by this liberal environment were not only numerous (secular) development organizations, but many organizations with political and religious agendas as well, creating anxiety among the political establishment and the population at large, and triggering calls for regulation. It soon became clear to the political elite that the challenge was to ensure that this emerging "civil society" would indeed remain "civil" and make a positive contribution to the common good. The government was particularly concerned about interethnic stability and cooperation, a sensitive topic because of recent clashes (in 1990) between Kyrgyz and Uzbeks and because of the "brain drain" of emigrating Russians and Germans. The topic became a central tenet of Akaev's political ideology, and was reflected in his slogan "Kyrgyzstan—our common home," which was meant to convey that all inhabitants of the republic, irrespective of their ethno-national and religious background, were an integral part of the newly independent country:

> I would propose the following philosophy. Your country is your home. Thus, our Kyrgyzstan is our common home. Indeed, it has been built by all of us, including Kyrgyz, Russians, Uzbeks, Germans, Jews, Uyghurs, Koreans, and Karachays. They built it without any doubt that they will live in this home as a single family in friendship and harmony, for eternity. (Akaev 1995, 97, in Murzakulova and Schoeberlein 2009, 1238)

This idea of a "common home" in which all nations contribute to the development of a harmonious society bears a strong resemblance to Soviet internationalism. As Asel Murzakulova and John Schoeberlein have pointed out, this was a "vision of a civic nation in the good traditions of the Soviet intelligentsia" (2009, 1238). In fact, ten years earlier Mikhail Gorbachev had used the exact same phrase to refer to the USSR.[6] But if Gorbachev had invoked "our common home" in order to smooth over ethnic tensions that erupted in the mid-1980s in the Caucasus and the Baltics especially, in Akaev's case there was an built-in tension. His internationalist references coincided with the particularistic effort of building an ethno-nation around the Kyrgyz majority, not least by elevating the mythical figure Manas as the key symbol of Kyrgyz nationhood.

Kyrgyzstan's secular leaders had expected that in the "postatheist" era, the return of religion would serve to strengthen the moral fabric of society and underpin the cultural historical traditions of the population. In one of his commentaries on the topic, Akaev summarized his views on the position of Islam in Kyrgyzstan as follows: "Here in Kyrgyzstan Islam was assimilated in a rather untraditional form. What we see here are the outward trappings of Islam without the exalted religious fanaticism and ideology. On the other hand, our brand of Islam absorbed many of the cultural traditions of the peoples in the region. . . . Our brand of Islam can play a stabilizing, consolidating role."[7] As we will see, however, this view was to be shaken as the years progressed, when it turned out that interest in "traditional" versions of Islam (and Christianity) remained subdued, while new religious movements quickly gained in importance and visibility.

It is important to remember the distinct spirit of optimism and possibility that existed in the early 1990s, as also David Lewis (2008) has observed. For a few years there was a real sense that things would improve quickly. In 1995, many of my acquaintances did not doubt that the transition to capitalism and democracy would be completed, even if they quibbled as to whether it would take five, ten, or as long as twenty years. But as time progressed, not only did the imagined endpoint recede further into the future, the country turned out to be moving in a very different direction. Despite economic liberalization, the anticipated (and promised) foreign investments never arrived. The loss of jobs was presented as a temporary setback, a side effect of the transition, but the reality was that stable formal employment remained rare even twenty-five years later. And although the Akaev government presented Kyrgyzstan as a "common home" for all nationalities, approximately half the population belonging to its minorities left the country for good.

One of the key problems with the economic reform programs, as also Janine Wedel has observed (2001), was that the Washington consensus did not sufficiently take into consideration the preexisting power relations, pretending instead that one can build a market economy through deregulation. Ignored were the tensions unleashed by privatization and the deep inequalities that the "free market" produced. And to assume that a cooperative heterogeneous population would emerge on the basis of an ideal of "international citizenship" was to ignore the tensions that afflict nation-state building. What thus needs to be analyzed is how former Soviet reality became refracted through the prism of the two grand narratives that were advanced in the 1990s and the 2000s: liberalism and nationalism. Crucially, the tropes of liberalism and nationalism became interwoven with the policies and laws of independent Kyrgyzstan, and affected how citizens experienced their own position in relation to the Kyrgyz state.

Privatization Chaos

When Kyrgyzstan embarked on a path of radical reform, the aim was to become an affluent market democracy in five to ten years. But while in the mid-1990s Kyrgyzstan counted as a hope-inspiring (neo-) liberal beacon in the region, twenty years later it had become an example of transition gone hopelessly wrong. Although it had been "doing everything right" from the perspective of the international community (Connery 2000, 4), the "shock therapy" strategy failed to attract major investors or result in sustainable economic growth. Poverty levels remained high despite a slow recovery in macroeconomic terms since the late 1990s; in 2003 real GDP was still only 78 percent of what it had been in 1989 (Pomfret 2006, 108). The accumulation of foreign debt during fifteen years of "transition" was staggering, to the extent that in 2006 the country met the criteria for access to the IMF and World Bank's Heavily Indebted Poor Countries Initiative. Two decades after gaining independence, Kyrgyzstan was at the bottom of former Soviet republics in terms of economic indicators, ranked among the most corrupt countries in the world, and had become politically volatile.

The reasons for this turn of events were many, but the most important ones can be illustrated by returning to the problematic assumptions of transition. Of the many critics of transition thinking, Thomas Carothers (2002) has been the most systematic in documenting the assumptions on which transition thinking was based, including, first, that the starting conditions and other specifics of "transitional countries" matter very little for the onset or the outcome of the transition process (8); second, that these transitions "are being built on coherent, functioning states" (8–9); and third, that fast reform is superior to gradual reform (see also Spoor 1995, 54, 61; Wedel 2001). The case of Kyrgyzstan dramatically illustrates the problems with these assumptions, which together demonstrate the fallacy of the overarching assumption, namely that "any country moving away from dictatorial rule can be considered a country in transition towards democracy" (Carothers 2002, 6), to eventually become a market democracy modeled on the North American example.

As has become more than obvious since, the starting conditions of individual countries have massively affected their post-Soviet trajectories. In fact, the economic prospects for an independent Kyrgyzstan had never been good. During Soviet times its economy had been based largely on agriculture and animal husbandry, coupled with coal and metallurgic mining activities as well as the production of components for the military industry. It lacked the natural riches of its neighbors such as oil and gas and had relied on a steady flow of subsidies from Moscow throughout the Soviet period. After independence, not only did the subsidies stop, but the mostly Russian markets for several of Kyrgyzstan's main commodities—meat, wool, machinery components, refined sugar—imploded with the disintegration of the Soviet Union. It is no big mystery why "transition countries" with close proximity to the European Union (such as the Baltic countries) fared considerably better, and why in the Central Asian context, the two countries that lacked substantial natural resources (Kyrgyzstan and Tajikistan) became not only the poorest post-Soviet republics but also the ones with the weakest state structures.

This brings us to the second point, the assumption that transition was built on functioning states. In reality, Kyrgyzstan's state system crumbled and fragmented under the weight of "transition." Talking about the upper echelons of Kyrgyz politics, Eric McGlinchey writes that "Kyrgyzstan's political mess is one of chaos" (2011, 2). He argues that because Kyrgyzstan lacked sufficiently large economic resources, the government was unable to buy the loyalty of its fragmented elite, resulting in considerable political instability (80–113). Actually, the problem extended far beyond the elite groups that McGlinchey focuses on. During much of the 1990s, the state was unable to pay its employees in health care, taxation, education, policing, and administration the kind of salaries that would meet minimum living costs, and often failed to pay out salaries for months on end. As Catherine Alexander (2009) has argued, for Kazakhstan in the 1990s this had the effect of the social contract coming undone, with the state losing its legitimacy. This resulting erosion of civil service was counteracted by a strengthening of informal ties, which increasingly personalized the state.

An interesting illustration of these processes is in Aksana Ismailbekova's book *Blood Ties and the Native Son* (forthcoming), which gives a detailed analysis of the political trajectory of Rahim, an aspiring leader in northern Kyrgyzstan. For Rahim to advance his political career the key issue is to extend his kinship-based support network by becoming regionally seen as a "native son," that is, as someone who will respectfully honor and reciprocate the support received from his home base. Perhaps ironically, these bonds of kinship and locality were solidified at moments that also symbolized capitalism and democracy: in the course of privatizing a factory, as the result of grants received from international development organizations, and especially on election days. Showing how these processes unfold in the context of "transition," Ismailbekova argues that kinship-based patronage practices should not be seen as the antithesis of democracy but rather as part of the development of a *vernacular democracy* with specific Kyrgyz features.

Finally, there is the issue of "fast" versus "gradual" reform. In Central Asia and more widely across the former Soviet Union, Kyrgyzstan counted as a fast reformer. But when in 1995 I talked with a group of Kyrgyz farmers about privatization, they told me: "If they [the government] would have privatized [all the assets] right away in 1991, we would have had thriving farms, but instead they waited, then they changed their minds, and in the meantime everything fell apart." These farmers were probably right in some respects, but the point is that a fast reform was never going to succeed in a situation in which the state system lacked the strength, coherence, and will to pull off a massive overnight transformation. Moreover, while the state system lacked willpower, the uncertainty and confusion about the direction of change fostered short-term rent seeking by those ordinary citizens and power holders with access to state resources. The result was catastrophic. As John Farrington (2005) documents, 57 percent of the livestock simply disappeared between 1989 and 1999.[8] Industrial production did not fare any better, with most of the (coal) mines and textile and food-processing factories closing their doors during the 1990s. In a situation where starting conditions are already unfavorable, and where the political structure lacks muscle to enforce its decisions, attempts at fast reforms are likely to be, in the words of Max Spoor (1995, 61) "hasty reforms" with disarticulating consequences.

In *The Anti-Politics Machine*, James Ferguson points out that development projects typically fail in reaching their objectives, in part because they are based on faulty assumptions and blueprints. Instead of focusing on failure, he proposes to focus on what failure produces, because, he says, "important political effects may be realized almost invisibly alongside . . . that 'failure' " (1990, 255). Analogously, we may ask: If in Kyrgyzstan neoliberal reform failed to produce a free market and a stable democracy, what did it produce instead? How was the political economy reconfigured as a result of neoliberal failure? It is important to keep in mind Joma Nazpary's observation that in Kazakhstan in the 1990s "privatization of state property [was] considered by the dispossessed as the root of chaos" (2002, 60). Beyond reflecting widespread frustration, this view rightly points at the affinities and interlinking of privatization, destabilization, and predatory accumulation. What had happened, in effect, was that economic liberalization allowed Soviet-rooted informal orders to assume new prominence and become the de facto regulating mechanisms.[9] Moreover, as the country entered a situation that depended on access to money rather than access to resources (Verdery 1996; Ledeneva 1998), Soviet forms of clientelism were transformed into post-Soviet "corruption," a process by which informal practices became monetized.

This dramatic development was, in many ways, the logical outcome of a poorly thought-out concept of "transition," which failed to acknowledge that political, economic, and other spheres of life are thoroughly interconnected, that therefore markets don't exist in vacuums, and indeed that "the economy" does not exist as an independent entity or separate sphere. The actual outcomes of "liberalization" could have been anticipated if "power" had been inserted into the equation. In fact, several prominent sociologists and anthropologists, most notably Caroline Humphrey (1991), Katherine Verdery (1996), and Michael Burawoy and Pavel Krotov (1992), very early on predicted that informal orders based on kinship, friendship, and locality would become the de facto ordering principles.

This turn of history was not entirely unanticipated within Kyrgyzstan either. Ironically, President Akaev seems to have been aware of the problems (as well as the possibilities for self-enrichment) even while upholding his image as a staunch believer in "transition" when he wrote in 1993 that the transition "has occurred somewhat illogically." Specifically, he noted that on the economic front "we enact economic freedom, while lacking developed property relations, primarily private property" (Akaev 1993). This illogicality, in a weak state, produced disastrous effect for the economy overall, while allowing well-placed political entrepreneurs (including Akaev) to appropriate large chunks of the economy.

This conjunction highlights the conceptual affinities between corruption and privatization. The classic definition of corruption as the "use of public office for private gain" may be reconfigured to hypothesize that the transformation of the public sector after socialism entailed an alternative mode of privatization—the "privatization of public offices and assets" by (groups of) well-placed individuals—without significantly changing the political culture, and without erasing existing networks of power. This process excluded the majority of citizens, while creating uncertainty for everyone (McGlinchey 2011; Shishkin 2013).[10] Ultimately, then, the Kyrgyz "transition" revealed in tragic detail how privatization and corruption feed on each other. Neoliberal policies had produced not an ideal-typical "free market" but rather, to use the local vocabulary, a "wild market" (*dikii rynok*).

Divisive Nationalism

In a landmark publication, Yuri Slezkine demolished the popular notion of the Soviet Union as a "breaker of nations" by documenting and boldly asserting that "Soviet nationality policy was devised and carried out by nationalists" (1994, 414). In the context of Central Asia's history, it is tempting to combine this perspective with the even bolder statement by Ernest Gellner that nationalism "invents nations where they do not exist" (1983). Indeed, in this region nations had not been in existence before the Russian Revolution. Its population had drawn lines of differentiation on the basis of religion, locality, tribal affiliation, language, and mode of livelihood, but these lines crosscut each other in numerous and often inconsistent ways and certainly did not congeal into coherent national categories. In fact, the labels "Kyrgyz," "Kazakh," "Uzbek," "Tadjik," and "Turkmen" were announced as national categories only in the 1920s, and they obtained substance in the decades that followed (Roy 2000, xvi).

The people who were categorized as Kyrgyz initially hardly identified with that label, referring to themselves primarily in terms of kinship, as member of a tribe or tribal segment, as pastoralists in contrast to the agriculturalists of the Fergana Valley, and as Muslims in contrast to the Russian administrators and settlers. But as Francine Hirsch (2005) and Olivier Roy (2000) have argued, by delineating ethno-territorial boundaries, developing administrative structures within those territories, and relegating power to local elites, the Soviet regime provided the incentives that infused ethno-national categories with a social and political life.[11] These categories gained further substance through the introduction of modern schooling in standardized national languages, and the promotion of cultural repertoires that included national cuisine, dress, music, and, in the case of the Kyrgyz, a national epic. As all successful inventions are, these were rooted in existing cultural material, but this was standardized and generalized to fit the needs of nationhood.

The national projects of the newly independent states were in many ways continuations of the nationality policies of the Soviet Union, while entering a context in which the supranational civic structure of the Union of Soviet Republics no longer existed. Indeed, after 1991 no one has seriously doubted the legitimacy of the five Soviet-produced Central Asian nations, nor were there serious attempts to create a pan-Turkistani state. When in 1991 Benedict Anderson wrote a new foreword to his famous book on the logics of nationalism, it may well have been that he had the new map of Central Asia in mind when stating that "history seems to be bearing out the 'logic' of *Imagined Communities* better than its author managed to do" ([1983] 2006, xi).

Though the Central Asian experience thus fits the general contours of the grand narrative of modern nationalism, the devil is in the details. Although these nations were either "invented" or solidified in the early twentieth century, this happened as part of the politics of the Soviet "affirmative action" empire (Martin 2001). That is, the national categories were produced before the territorial units to which they corresponded gained their own independent political life. Moreover, because of the (unavoidable) incongruence between territorial divisions and ethno-national categories (and because of the forced and voluntary labor migrations), each newly independent post-Soviet country contained significant preformed minorities with their own designated homelands elsewhere. The Kyrgyz SSR is a case in point. In the last Soviet census, of 1989, only a slight majority, 52 percent, of its population was classified as ethnically Kyrgyz (Anderson 1999, 42). Additionally, the republic was home to a large contingent of Russians (21%) and Uzbeks (13%), as well as many smaller minorities, of which Tatars, Uyghurs, Germans, and Ukrainians were the most numerous.

These ethno-national categories gained new significance when the overarching Soviet civic administrative structure made way for sovereign national territories, often with negative consequences for minorities. As Rogers Brubaker has pointed out, while the age of nationalism appeared to be drawing to a close in other parts of the world, post-Soviet Eurasia was "moving back to the nation-state, entering not a post-national but a post-multinational era" (2011, 1786). To draw attention to the incompleteness of the nation-state project Brubaker proposes to speak instead of "nationalizing states" (2011). This is a useful perspective because even though the "nations" remained uncontested in the geopolitical arena, at the subnational level they competed with other frames of belonging. In Kyrgyzstan there was considerable tension between national, regional, and tribal components of collective ideology.[12]

To illustrate these tensions it makes sense to return to the Manas epic and its hero, Batyr-khan Manas, whom we already encountered in the form of his statue. The epic had been treated with ambivalence by Soviet authorities, alternately being denounced as reactionary and celebrated as representative of native culture, in which case it was presented as "expressing the deepest moral aspirations of the masses" and reflecting the "working conditions of the people" (van der Heide 2008, 182–83). Plans to celebrate the epic's thousand-year existence had been made since the 1930s, but were postponed time and again, most likely because the epic revolves around warfare between the Kyrgyz and Chinese-speaking Kalmyk tribes, a diplomatically sensitive issue. However, as soon as Kyrgyzstan declared independence, Manas was promoted as the cornerstone of the government's nationalizing efforts, and his one-thousandth anniversary was celebrated in 1995. Manas came to be presented as "the embodiment of the Kyrgyz self-image" (Thompson et al. 2006, 178), and the epic as a model for moral and spiritual guidance to the Kyrgyz nation (van der Heide 2008, 272; Marat 2008). Schoolchildren were taught the seven lessons of Manas: patriotism, unity of the nation, international cooperation, defense of the state, humanism, harmony with nature, and the aspiration to obtain knowledge and skills (Akaev 2003, 420–24). Celebrated narrators of the epic (*manaschis*) were given prominent places in the new pantheon of national heroes. A flood of popular publications and public events further helped elevate the epic to the standing of a national ideology.

Notwithstanding the substantial strengths of Manas as a national symbol, he also revealed cracks in the state-building effort. The first tension was that the principle of "genealogical relatedness" on which Manas worship was built did as much to divide the Kyrgyz into tribes as unite them as a nation (Gullette 2010). The figure of Manas, whose place of birth and death is believed to have been in the Talas Valley in northwestern Kyrgyzstan, found more resonance in the north of the country than in the south, where the epic and its hero had never played a prominent role. The second tension was that as an ethno-national mythological hero, the figure of Manas implicitly excluded all non-Kyrgyz, thereby reinforcing the notion that ultimately Kyrgyzstan is the home of the ethnic Kyrgyz rather than for its substantial non-Kyrgyz population.

The government was all too aware of the gravity of these issues. In the period between 1989 and 1999 the Russian population in Kyrgyzstan decreased by 313,000 (from 916,000 to 603,000), which represented a drop from 21.5 to 12.5 percent of the total population. In addition, some 58,000 Ukrainians and 80,000 Germans left the Kyrgyz Republic, mostly in the early 1990s. This exodus was particularly problematic because it constituted a significant brain drain, as Russians and other "Europeans"[13] were more likely to have completed higher education and were strongly represented in the technical, managerial, and educational spheres. Although economic factors formed the main reason for this massive emigration (prospects were not good in Kyrgyzstan), it was also the case that many "Europeans" did not feel at home in an independent Kyrgyzstan, where the Kyrgyz language was replacing Russian as the main administrative language and where careers were increasingly dependent on being part of networks that followed lines of ethnicity and kinship (Kosmarskaia 2006).

Akaev tried to counteract these tensions during his presidency, from 1991 to 2005, by stressing the integrative elements of Manas, and the applicability of his wisdom to humanity as a whole. This is a recurring theme in his book *Kyrgyz Statehood and the National Epos "Manas,"* in which he writes that a key idea of the epic is "transethnic consensus, friendship, and cooperation" (Akaev 2003, 283). Moreover, through his slogan "Kyrgyzstan—our common home" that we have encountered earlier, Akaev stressed that the Kyrgyz nation should be seen as a "polyethnic alloy," one that is stronger than the "initial materials" (2003, 32). According to Murzakulova and Schoeberlein, this kind of recycling of "Soviet internationalism" was meant to suggest continuity with the Soviet past and to appeal to Kyrgyzstan's minorities, especially Russians, while the government's use of nationalist symbolism was aimed at pleasing the Kyrgyz majority population. Both aspects were, according to the authors, aimed at obtaining "the solidarity and loyalty of different groups within the state and when one of them does not function, the other is deployed" (Murzakulova and Schoeberlein 2009, 1239). Although tensions remained, this two-track approach served the goals of simultaneously legitimizing power and softening the anxieties of minorities.

Things changed after the Tulip Revolution of 2005. As Madeleine Reeves points out, while President Akaev's slogans had celebrated Kyrgyzstan as a common home for a multiethnic population, Bakiev's rhetoric emphasized "patriarchal values and deference to political authority" (2014b, 69). In other words, while during Akaev's presidency the government still used inclusive rhetoric to appeal to Uzbeks, Russians, and others, the absence of a civic ideology under Bakiev and more frequent use of nationalist rhetoric heightened the sense of insecurity among Uzbeks and other minorities (Cummings 2012, 86).

As mentioned above, attempts to create a civic nation rooted in a Soviet internationalist ideal had never been entirely successful. They had gone hand in hand with policies and a reimagining of the nation with which non-Kyrgyz were hardly able to identify. In northern Kyrgyzstan, most Russians who were able to return to Russia did so because they no longer saw a future. The ethnic composition was different in the south. There, the substantial Uzbek minority had never migrated to Kyrgyzstan, but had ended up on the wrong side of the border when the administrative boundaries between Soviet Socialist Republics were delineated in the 1930s. During the Soviet period this did not matter very much, and the Uzbek part of the population of the Kyrgyz SSR had oriented itself to the cities in Uzbekistan, where many followed secondary education and found marriage partners. These connections were maintained after the collapse of the Soviet Union, but this also meant that the Uzbek minority in Kyrgyzstan was caught between states' borders, occupying a marginal position with regard to both countries (Liu 2012, 44).

To sum up, the ethno-national categories that were fixed and fastened through Soviet classificatory processes reflected previously existing lines of differentiation in economic activities, settlement patterns, and marital relationships. But the categories had long been fluid and permeable, and continued to be so during the Soviet period. The categories Kyrgyz and Uzbek were infused with new relevance, however, after the demise of the multinational Soviet state. In conditions of uncertainty and fragmentation, the national categories achieved affective qualities that rendered them salient as a mobilizing force, around which ideas of "the people" could be rallied. During particular episodes this allowed for an intensification of "groupness" (Brubaker 2004)—a surge of populist nationalism, with destructive tendencies.

Volatility in a Weak State

On the morning of June 10, 2010, as I was sitting in a Bishkek office, news started to pour in about clashes between Kyrgyz and Uzbeks in the southern city of Osh. I discussed the news with Elmira, the office secretary. At that point we knew very little about what was happening, but she was certain that things would remain quiet in the capital: "In the south they have a different mentality; here [in the capital] people are more civilized and educated." Over the next twenty-four hours the conflict spread from Osh to several other towns in the south, including Jalalabad and Bazar-Korgon, two places I had previously lived and had many friends and acquaintances. I was on the phone with young Uzbek men from Bazar-Korgon who had tried to escape into Uzbekistan only to find the border gates closed to them. I talked to an Uzbek mother of an all-female household who was terrified, as she was listening to the approaching gunfire (which luckily never reached her street). I phoned a Kyrgyz acquaintance in Kokjangak who mentioned that, even though there were clashes in nearby Jalalabad (a mere thirty kilometers away), he was certain that nothing would happen where he lived because the mixed population in this former mining town had long been accustomed to interacting civilly across ethnic lines.

The conflict raged for three days, leaving hundreds of people dead, 80 percent of whom were Uzbek, and thousands of houses burned.[14] More than one hundred thousand women and children temporarily fled to Uzbekistan, and approximately three hundred thousand people were internally displaced (Kyrgyzstan Inquiry Commission 2011). The police and military had done very little to stop the violence, and in some instances actively aided Kyrgyz attackers, thereby significantly contributing to the destructive force of the conflict (International Crisis Group 2010). Mass violence did not spread to Bishkek, but for about a week people in the capital lived in fear, with streets left deserted in the evenings, the territory of young men with cars, ghetto blasters, and booze.

Since the mid-2000s Kyrgyzstan has experienced a series of tumultuous political events, of which the two revolutions, of March 2005 and April 2010, and the above-described bloodshed between Kyrgyz and Uzbeks in June 2010 were the most dramatic ones. The Tulip Revolution of 2005 started after fraudulent elections had left several opposition leaders out of parliament, creating unrest among significant factions of the political elite, which then started to merge with the frustrations of ordinary citizens about a "transition" that was going nowhere. Still, no one expected that the protests, which initially seemed a provincial affair, would travel so quickly to the capital and remove Akaev from power with so little resistance. As one of the main opposition leaders (and the later president) Kurmanbek Bakiev reportedly exclaimed: "We did not expect this at all. It was not part of the plan."[15] The sudden breakdown of state structures set the stage for several chaotic days in the capital, but a sense of calm returned after two days.

The background to the second Kyrgyz revolution, of April 2010, was frustration about the cronyism and predatory practices of the Bakiev regime. Frustration culminated with several increases in energy prices, which were blamed on the malversations of the presidential family, and after which people in the provinces started attacking government offices. In contrast to Akaev in 2005, Kurmanbek Bakiev and his family did not leave without a fight, resulting in clashes that left eighty-six people dead (Matveeva 2010). In the chaos that followed the April 2010 revolution several instances of intercommunal violence erupted, of which the earlier described June 2010 conflict between Kyrgyz and Uzbeks was the most devastating.

These two revolutions as well as the 2010 bloodshed have been much commented on.[16] Not only have these events been constitutive of the political landscape and should thus be prominently discussed in a contextual chapter, they also powerfully illuminate the affective dimension of politics. Though each revolution had been long in coming, when actual fighting broke out, it took people by surprise. Through these dramatic events, rooted in messy realities, certainty was being produced. Indeed, it was during the days of conflict that the contours of "imagined communities" achieved frightening clarity (McBrien 2013, 259–60). And it was during the 2010 revolution that the notion of "the people" gained crucial importance (Reeves 2014b). In these events the slow-paced ideological shifts were interrupted by fast-paced contentious politics.

It is not difficult to see how these dramatic political events were rooted in the murkiness of the "transition." The last years of Akaev's rule were characterized by dwindling hope that the transition would ever be completed. Kyrgyz society had been descending into a negative spiral of instability and anomie. Increasing frustration with the regime started to intertwine with the frustrations of important segments of the political elite. The years after the Tulip Revolution revealed a further worsening of the situation. Protests that focused on price hikes, administrative incompetence, and imprisonment of politicians had become commonplace in the capital as well as in the provinces. Tensions along ethnic lines became more visible (Tabyshalieva 2013) and often focused on land entitlements. Administrative offices had increasingly become dominated by Kyrgyz (and organized along regional and tribal lines), a process that intensified after 2005, thereby further marginalizing minority groups.

Even if in hindsight it is clear that the dramatic events were rooted in a failed transition, at the moment they happened everyone was taken aback. Ironically, even the leaders of the Tulip Revolution commented that they had not planned for revolution. And regarding the clashes of 2010, Julie McBrien argues that "no one imagined and no one anticipated the violence" (2013, 257). One reason is people's tendency to distance themselves from violence and turmoil, preferring to attribute them to barbarism or uncivilized behavior (as in Elmira's dismissal). Another reason is that the triggers that set off dramatic chains of events were seemingly minor: electoral fraud in 2005 (such fraud had happened before); a hike in energy tariffs in 2010 (painful but one in a row of hikes); a fight between young men (once again).[17] What happened in each of these cases, however, was that these small triggers started to reverberate with other frustrations, fears, and anxieties. Within an already fragmented political landscape, these incidents symbolized a broken space that separated people from power, feeding into a "constitutive antagonism" (Laclau 2005, 85) that provided the impetus for group mobilization and radicalization.

In the case of the conflict between Kyrgyz and Uzbeks, the anxieties of the Kyrgyz majority were fueled by Uzbek calls for emancipation. Indeed, in the period leading up to the conflict, the "politically marginalized Uzbek minority had become increasingly involved in regional and national politics, and had made more vocal demands for equal treatment and opportunities" (McBrien 2011, 3). This was perceived in some Kyrgyz circles as an affront to the country's sovereignty, imagined as an "ethno-national and popular institution," as David Gullette and John Heathershaw (2015, 125) have pointed out. In the case of the 2005 Tulip Revolution the trigger was electoral fraud, which started to resonate with the suspicion that Akaev was consolidating the influence of the presidential family on the national political scene. Moreover, these practices were uncovered at a time when opposition newspapers published images of some of the family's spacious residences along with a list of companies that belonged to, or were controlled by, the Akaev family. Outrage about these practices played an important role in the unrest—numerous reports noted that protesters were driven by a sense that Akaev and his family had "gone too far."[18] In the 2010 revolution it was the combination of the announced rise in energy prices together with the sentiment that the Bakiev family's greed had spun out of control.[19]

The trigger, far from being trivial, creates a focal point around which discourse "thickens" as it reverberates with accumulated resentment and frustration, which then becomes tied to the aspirations of temporarily marginalized elites, thereby kicking in a new and semiautonomous dynamic of violence. As Bruce Kapferer has argued, it is during conflict that political myths—fantasies of purity, justice, or supremacy—become "imbued with commanding power" (1988, 47). In a similar vein the 2010 revolution served to crystallize "the people" (*el*) versus the government, and moreover, as Reeves (2014b) astutely notices, the notion of "the people" obtained exclusivist ethnic Kyrgyz connotations, paving the way for episodes of violence against non-Kyrgyz minorities in the months ahead.

In Bishkek in the months after the April 2010 revolution a standard joke was that while other democracies have elections every four or five years, Kyrgyzstan has a revolution every five years. But whereas one could make jokes about corrupt politicians, and perhaps even celebrate the people's ability to remove corrupt autocrats from power, similar jokes did not exist about the ethnic conflicts that occurred in 1990 and 2010 between

Kyrgyz and Uzbeks. Don Kalb argues in his (2005) article "From Flows to Violence" that market-led development programs have destabilizing effects. In Kyrgyzstan, political turmoil was rooted in a disastrous transition that left people frustrated and hollowed out the state, becoming a shell to be captured and mobilized by rotating factions. In this fragile environment, seemingly small triggers could set in motion chains of action and reaction with transformative potential, but often resulting in further disillusionment and astonishment about the fragility of order. As one of my friends from Bazar-Korgon told me: "I had never expected that [these atrocities] would happen *here*, in *our* town." But those violent events did occur, producing temporary clarity about who is friend and who is foe, yet blurring the future.

Lenin's Shadow

> I'm afraid that I don't really know what capitalism means. I conceive of it as the development in the West. When someone uses the word "capitalism" I think about the United States. I think of a highly developed industrialized country. At the moment, Kyrgyzstan is moving in the direction of capitalism in all spheres of life. I don't know what this means. We have a wild market and perhaps that is a first step on the road to capitalism, [but] I don't think that Kyrgyzstan will become a capitalist country very soon.

These sentences were written by an undergraduate student at the Issyk Kul State University in northeastern Kyrgyzstan in 1995, after I had asked her and fifteen fellow students to write take-home essays on the topic of capitalism. Several students copied or paraphrased the contents of Soviet encyclopedias and/or their parents' opinion, such as one who said that "capitalism is the socioeconomic structure that is based on private property and the exploitation of people," and another that "money is the dominant factor in capitalism. You can buy everything with money, even labor force. People are divided into poor (the laborers) and rich (the capitalists)." Ironically, these lines described the post-Soviet reality of the times quite accurately. However, even the students who employed such communist language ended their essays in ways that radically departed from a communist or socialist perspective. The last-quoted student, for example, continued by writing that "although capitalism still has these and other problems [referring to poverty and inequality], I do think that it is a good system. After all, many of the highly developed countries have a form of capitalism." Taken together, the essays appeared to reflect "minds in transition," in which the dominant theme was hope that the problems would be overcome and that the country was treading a path toward prosperity. In the words of one student, "Our country will become civilized and people won't be unemployed, but will instead work hard and receive high wages."

What struck me in these essays was the students' ability to continue believing in a future affluent society despite living in increasingly impoverished conditions. And crucially, the essays suggested two mechanisms for how such hope could be maintained. The first involved denial that capitalism had already "arrived," by stating instead that their society was "moving in the direction" or was still only in the "first stage" of what was going to be capitalism, and that this would ultimately replace the despised "wild market." This response was understandable as the reality they experienced was radically different from the capitalism that they imagined to exist in "highly developed industrial societies." This, moreover, points to the second mechanism, which was to imagine capitalism as a return of the state. Inherent in the dismissal of the "wild market" was the idea that the market would be tamed by a proactive government. Similar sentiments surfaced when I talked (we are still in 1995) with a teacher who had not been paid his salary for months, yet who did not consider becoming an entrepreneur a viable option:

> If I would give up this job and become a trader, I would end up with nothing. At the bazaar there are no pensions. And what happens when you get ill? When everything goes back to normal in a few years, those traders will be empty-handed: without work, without money, without anything!

As empty signifiers (Laclau 1993) capitalism and democracy were able to signal the impending arrival of affluent society. Many conceptualized capitalism as a better functioning version of socialism, and only gradually realized that the welfare state they had lost was not going to come back.

In the two decades that have passed since 1995, the "return to normal" never happened. In the end, the kind of advanced capitalism that could guarantee affluence for most people did not develop, nor did the state step back in to reign in exploitation and provide a safety net for its weaker citizens. Liberal ideology did not come with a concrete vision of how to reorder society but closely followed the Washington consensus, which amounted to privatizing the state, a process favoring the well-endowed and well positioned, while leaving the majority of residents scrambling for survival. It produced a volatile situation ruled by money, one ordered along unstable lines of clientelism and patronage. When in the early 2010s my acquaintances reflected on the 1990s they would speak of hardship and confusion and emphasize that they had been in shock. But they would also say that the present was not much different; they had simply gotten used to their chaotic lives.

Although from an outsider's perspective the neoliberal shift of the 1990s had objectively constituted a "passing of mass utopia" (Buck-Morss 2000), it took a while for this realization to set in. This was not in small measure due to the fact that "capitalism" and "democracy" were powerful empty signifiers that perpetuated hope, meanwhile narrowing political debate and thereby legitimizing the Akaev government. As such it was a convenient cover, or mask, for a reconfiguration of politics and economy that went on behind the scenes. Given the discrepancy between neoliberal rhetoric and chaotic reality, it was only a matter of time, though, for this mask to be revealed for what it was and for "transition" to come unstuck.

This unraveling of transition does not mean there are no utopian projects left. Rather, the downfall of the hegemonic state machinery for the production and distribution of hope produced anxieties and fears (cf. Hage 2003, 3), while providing a boost to other hope-generating mechanisms and movements. The shattered transition not only destabilized economic lives but also opened up a space in which a range of ideological movements could thrive. It was because of this that evangelical Pentecostals talked about Kyrgyzstan as a "ripe harvest field" (cited in Pelkmans 2006b, 29); and Islamic piety movements such as the Tablighi Jamaat saw Kyrgyzstan as a "clean slate," and were able to connect with the sensibilities of young Muslim men (as discussed in chapter 4). Hence, the post-Soviet condition is more appropriately described as one of ideological excess than ideological void (Borenstein 1999). But this ideological excess, which refers to the conspicuous presence of nationalist, market, developmental, and religious visions, also suggests the fragility of each single ideology.

With the passing of two decades, the dream of a capitalist future of abundance turned out to be a mirage that could never be reached, while the memory of socialist security and order receded into the past. The images of abundance and safety never disappeared but were reconfigured to become part of other ideologies, or indeed lingered on in the thoughts of those living through hardship. For now, let me give just one example, of a woman in her fifties who was fighting back her tears when we talked in 2013 in her flat in the small former mining town of Ak-Tiuz. Ever since she had lost her job eighteen years previously she had retained some hope that eventually she would be able to work again as a nurse. She was hopeful when, earlier that year, a Canadian company was recruiting a nurse to be based in her small town (not least because she was the only resident with an education in nursing), but in the interview she was told that her experience was out-of-date. A young woman from a neighboring town was hired instead. Angrily she said that in the past employers would have always looked first at whether locally skilled labor was available: "back then they cared about the community." True or not, Mirgul's hopes had been informed by how labor used to be organized in former times, a coalescing of the past and the future in the present that resulted in despair.

Lenin used to adorn not only Ala-Too Square but countless other squares throughout the country. These provincial Lenins do not have the same allure, but they have equally interesting things to say about the course of history. In post-Soviet Kyrgyzstan most of these Lenins remained in place even when their surroundings radically altered. A good example is the Lenin that stood in front of the entrance of the tool-parts factory in Kokjangak. The factory went bankrupt, the buildings were dismantled, and the construction materials sold, leaving behind nothing but a field of concrete waste. But in the middle of this rubble, Lenin was still standing. I cannot say if this Lenin's survival was deliberate, but another Lenin in the same town suggested that this might well have been the case. This other Lenin had been standing in front of the city hall. When, in 2002, he was moved away from the entrance to be repositioned nearby, his legs accidentally broke off. Instead of discarding the maimed statue, a cast was built around Lenin's legs, such that it would look as if he was leaning over a wall.

It is tempting to interpret this treatment as an act of "restorative nostalgia" (Boym 2001), but the people I asked about it were evasive, presenting

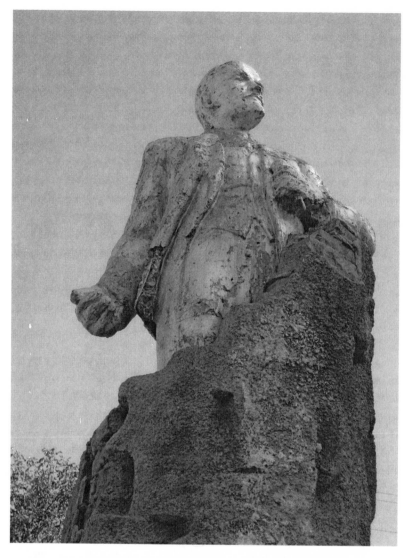

The patched-up Lenin statue in the center of Kokjangak, August 2009

it as an artistic innovation or making jokes about their wobbly Lenin. Whether or not this Lenin offered comfort or acted as an anchor in lives of turmoil, destroying Lenin or leaving him injured would clearly have been inappropriate.

If these stories reflect nostalgia for a past in which there was order and purpose, a final Lenin story brings out the ambivalent aspects of this relationship with the past. Beside the main road in Ak-Tiuz, near the town hall, stands a silver-painted statue of Lenin. At first sight there is nothing remarkable about this Lenin; it is one of the "standard" Lenins, one in which he brings his left hand up to his chest while looking into the distance as if addressing an audience. But what is striking about this particular statue is that it bears saw marks—horizontal lines cut into his chest, waist, knees, and ankles. Reportedly, some men had made the cuts in order to find out whether Lenin's insides contained anything of value, but on discovering that his insides contained nothing but air and concrete, they didn't proceed with dismantling the statue. In its wounded guise, the statue appears symbolic of the ways in which past, present, and future have come together. In the Soviet past, the future was present in slogans and plans pointing to a utopian communism. However, this utopian vision turned out to be quite hollow when the Soviet Union started to descend, just as the statue turned out to be worthless when attacked with a saw.

And yet the hollow Lenin is still standing, twenty-four years after the demise of the Soviet Union. Lenin was no longer revered, and yet there was no symbol to replace him with. This in itself could be taken as indicative of the weakness of the state, and of the fragility of the new ideologies that were being advanced. Just like in so many other locations, there was no lack of visions for the future—in fact there was an excess of them—but their institutional backing was weak or absent, and many people had become doubtful of their promises of a better future. The turmoil of ideas that swept through Kyrgyzstan showed the fragility of each ideological vision, which in any case only addressed a part of the population. By contrast, even though Soviet implementation used to be chaotic (Kotkin 1995) and produced many excesses, its vision of a better future remained unwavering. Perhaps it was for this reason that this Lenin was patched up. His cuts were smoothed over and given a new lick of paint in 2014. What the fate of these Lenin statues appeared to signify was not so much nostalgia for a past that was lost as nostalgia for hope in a better future.

2

Condition of Uncertainty

Life in an Industrial Wasteland

A middle-aged Kyrgyz man, dressed in worn-out clothes, was walking
through the park, looking around with apparent incredulity. He noticed me
sitting in the shade of a tree, and called out: "What is this place? This looks
like Afghanistan. It's one fucking war zone." We had a short conversation.
"I used to live here," he explained, "but everything has vanished. I still
recognize the park because it has Lenin standing over there, but that's all."
He had returned (in 2008) after an absence of almost twenty years, having
worked in construction throughout Russia. On his last assignment, just after
he and his working party had started on a construction project in Sochi, his
possessions, including his passport, were stolen. Left with just a minimal
sum, he had barely made it back to the hometown he no longer recognized.

Between 1960 and 1990 Kokjangak had approximately twenty thousand
inhabitants, many of whom worked in the coal mine (up to four thousand employees) and the sewing and radio-parts factories (together fifteen
hundred employees). But with the scaling down and eventual closure of
the mine and factories after the collapse of the USSR, half its population
moved away, until stabilizing at around ten thousand by the late 1990s.[1]
Kokjangak came to be known as one of the poorest settlements in Jalalabad Province, a town where the remaining population struggled to make
ends meet. They mixed small-scale urban-based agriculture and animal
husbandry with informal mining activities and jobs in the service sector,
and relied to a significant degree on state benefits and remittances sent by
relatives working in Russia.

Amid these overwhelming changes the only constant appeared to be uncertainty. The crumbling of the socialist welfare state and the unwieldiness of the "wild market" economy had the effect that inhabitants could neither rely on state provisions nor be confident that their private initiatives paid off. This "post-Soviet chaos" (Nazpary 2002) should not, however, be understood as the absence of order but rather as a structured disorder that allowed for predatory accumulation by those in power.[2] The residents shared this predicament with most other ordinary citizens of Kyrgyzstan, who all experienced the painful postsocialist "transition," the destabilizing effects of two revolutions, and continuing political instability. But in Kokjangak this uncertainty was exacerbated by the unraveling of social networks (due to massive outmigration) and the complete disappearance of industry. The uncertainties were intricately connected to the decaying urban landscape. As inhabitants projected their frustrations, fears, and hopes onto their surroundings, the landscape impressed itself onto them, meshing with existential and ontological concerns.

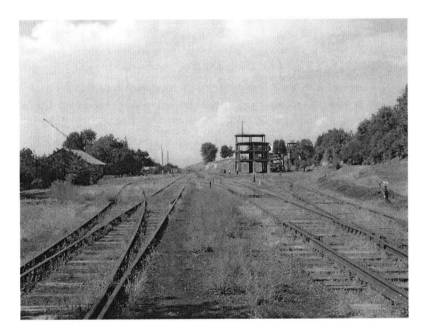

Abandoned train tracks leading to the former coal mine in Kokjangak, July 2008

Residents who continued to live in Kokjangak through the 1990s may never have experienced the sudden shock of bewilderment expressed by the returnee quoted above; yet the city's downfall continued to confront everyone who had known Kokjangak in its Soviet glory. Residents were reminded of those better times on a daily basis when passing the remainders of what once were buildings, or when dealing with the absence of drinkable tap water, garbage disposal, and public transportation. In conversation they used indicators of places that had ceased to exist: they said "behind the office building [*za kontoroi*]" when referring to the coal mine's headquarters, where nothing but the concrete foundations remained; "near the bus station [*vozle avtovokzala*]" referred to a place from which no bus had departed since the mid-1990s. When they described their city to outsiders, key words included "war zone," "devastation," and "death." Kokjangak was a "dying city" (*umeraiushchii gorod*) or, in the words of a newspaper reporter, a "lifeless stokehole" (*potukhshaia kochegarka*).[3] To add insult to injury, in the early 2000s Kokjangak was administratively reclassified, losing its status of "city" (*gorod*) to become a "settlement of urban type" (*poselok gorodskogo tipa*).

Aiming to capture the process of decline, an article titled "Dying City" in the national newspaper *Vechernii Bishkek* wrote about Kokjangak: "It is not difficult to destroy a city. There is no need even to bomb it. All that is needed is to take away hope and belief in tomorrow. Then the city will destroy itself."[4] It is worthwhile to reflect for a moment on this presumed absence of hope. Certainly, people's dwindling confidence in the future revival of their town played a role in their decision to leave. Kokjangak was a "dying city," a postindustrial wasteland, a ruin of Soviet modernity. Its entire territory was covered with scars—reminders of a different and better past, of the pain of recent rupture, and of the struggle to survive. And yet, seemingly paradoxically but also logically, the hopelessness of the situation and the collapse of grand ideology generated renewed hope and triggered the appearance of new ideological visions. As Jarrett Zigon has rightly argued, hope is not the product of good times but arises in conditions of struggle (2009, 262). Moreover, it can never completely free itself from that struggle. "Hope can never be fully divorced from hopelessness any more than hopelessness can be divorced from hope" (Crapanzano 2004, 114); they drive each other on and are in constant risk of slippage.[5]

In this chapter, then, I examine both the absence of ideology and its hesitant return, offering a meditation on hopeless situations and the concomitant glimmering of hope. By focusing on the inhabitants of a destitute former mining town and urban wasteland, I aim to understand how political-economic transformation and urban decline affect how people engage with the big questions of existence: How to survive? What to do? Who and what to trust? What to believe? As we will see, in this instance the condition of uncertainty produced an apparent openness to new ideologies, yet an openness that was coupled with reticence, a curiosity matched with suspicion, all of which resonated with the landscape.

(Pre-)Historic Sketch

The name "Kokjangak" literally means "blue-green nut" and refers to the modest walnut forest that once covered most of the uphill valley where the city was built. Residents praised the location's climatic features; located on a southern slope of the Ala-Too Mountains it is protected from the cold northern winds in winter, whereas its elevated location (between 1,200 and 1,400 meters) means that summers are not as hot as in the basin of the Suzak Valley (which is a branch of the Fergana Valley). In the early twentieth century the hills belonged, according to the Osmonov family tradition, to their grandfather Osman, who had been given the land by a powerful *bey* in appreciation of provided services. Some years later, however, he had to tolerate the presence of Russian explorers (geologists). Osman's contempt for and distrust of these Russians reputedly was such that he forbade his children to talk to them or eat their "heathen bread," and eventually he moved his household a kilometer downstream to what is now the neighborhood *kölmö* (the Kyrgyz word for *sovkhoz*, state farm).[6]

Coal-mining activities started in the 1910s (Kashirin 1988) but were interrupted after the Russian Revolution and the ensuing struggle for power (1918–22) between Bolsheviks and Basmachis, with the latter allegedly responsible for blowing up the mine.[7] Mining activities expanded in the second half of the 1920s. A Russian communist who was sent to Kokjangak to organize labor reported that in 1927 there were "approximately seventy miners who extracted the coal with primitive means, primarily by hand," and who in their free time would carry out voluntary work to speed up the development of the town (quoted in Chormonov and Sidorov 1963, 102).[8] Urban development accelerated after Kokjangak became connected to the provincial city of Jalalabad by train tracks and a gravel road in 1932. By 1939 Kokjangak had developed into a sizable town with eight thousand inhabitants, of which 1,009 were employed in the mine (ibid., 123, 129).

As elsewhere in the Soviet empire, the rapid urbanization and industrialization of the Stalinist era were accompanied by coercion, severe shortages, and other excesses (cf. Kotkin 1995; Fitzpatrick 1999). The plateau just above the city center is a reminder of this coercive past. Called *Zona* (the zone), it refers to the labor camp that was located there until the 1960s. It had been created for German prisoners of war and was subsequently used for other convicts, both categories of which were deployed in labor-intensive infrastructural projects. People who came to Kokjangak on their own accord during the 1930s and 1940s encountered conditions that were hardly more favorable. An elderly Kyrgyz man told me: "When they arrived, there often was not even a place for them to sleep. During the first nights many ended up sleeping on the warm coal waste, but this was warm because [poisonous] gas was still burning inside. One morning twenty dead bodies were found. All had died in their sleep." Despite such tragedies, moving to town was often preferable to the impoverished life in the villages: in Kokjangak, at least, "they paid workers in products and in money."

The same man also spoke to me about the arrival of deportees from the Caucasus, mostly Kurds and Chechens, and the ensuing tensions with the established population:

> They are also Muslim, but they are different. They wouldn't sleep at night. Instead they roamed around, stealing our cattle and other possessions. We tolerated it for a while, but then one night our men gathered, mounted their horses, took clubs with them, and beat up [the Chechens]. That was justified, because back then there weren't enough men around to protect each household—so we had to teach them a lesson.

Built on a foundation of coercion and tension, Kokjangak gained city status (it became a *gorod*) in 1943 and retained its position as a small yet regionally important industrial city throughout the Soviet period. Mining towns such as Kokjangak were purposely designed as *modern* socialist cities, showcases of Soviet progress, as described in the following text about the history of mining in the Kyrgyz SSR:

> Former poverty-stricken mining settlements transformed into comfortable and well-equipped [*blagoustroennye*] socialist cities . . . which please the eye with their multilevel architectural ensembles, their paved [asphalted] roads, green gardens and parks, their houses of culture, schools, stadiums, and much else that beautifies the miner's life [*byt*]. (Chormonov and Sidirov 1963, 162–63)

This description captures the Kokjangak that continued to occupy the collective imagination after its demise—a modern city with a diverse population, with abundant work in its coal mine and factories. Stories about these heydays will feature throughout this chapter, but the following (slightly edited) excerpt from a document produced by the city administration in the year 2000 offers a usefully detailed reflection of this image of modern urbanity:

> The city of Kokjangak has a developed infrastructure for electrical power, a communal hot water and central heating system, drinking water supply and a sewage system. . . . There are four post offices with sixteen employees providing telecommunication services. . . . The House of Culture, built in 1948, has a capacity for 600 visitors. . . . There is also a disco-club, a cinema called *shakter* [miner] and a city radio broadcasting center. . . . The city newspaper *Kokjangak Kabarlary* has a circulation of a 1,000 copies. A children's recreational center called *Barchyn* is located two kilometres outside the city and was constructed in 1976. It has eighty beds and is visited annually by about 250 children in three shifts. There is a central city stadium, built in 1958, with capacity for 2,000 spectators. (http://www.citykr.kg/en/kokjangak.php)

In short, Kokjangak had everything that one might expect of a small Soviet industrial city. But reading these features described in the present tense in a document written long after the USSR collapsed is surreal, not only because some of these modern features come across as anachronistic, but also because many of the services and venues had either stopped working or ceased to exist. As the document proceeds:

> The House of Culture requires a complete overhaul and renovation of its equipment. . . . The city printing house no longer operates due to the

deterioration of the printing presses. . . . The children's recreational center has not functioned in the last two years. . . . 1,500m³ of solid waste have accumulated over several years, which creates the conditions for the spread of infectious diseases. (www.citykr.kg/en/kokjangak.php)

The list could have been longer, because the mentioned cinema and disco-club had been reduced to rubble, the stadium had become pastureland for cows, and the central heating system was no longer able to heat the schools let alone the apartment buildings that also used to be connected to the system. When I first visited Kokjangak in 1998, the contours of the modern Soviet city were still distinctly visible, but they rapidly faded in subsequent years.

By 2008 the Soviet past had become a chimera, with even returnees failing to recognize their hometown. In the context of such encompassing transformation, in which the city's infrastructure had collapsed and half its population had left for good, the connections between past and present were tenuous. Kokjangak was a city that was being undone. Even the documents detailing its history had vanished. When I asked the mayor about the books, reports, and newspapers produced in and about Soviet Kokjangak, he told me, only partly in jest, that these had all disappeared in toilets. Whether this was literally true or not, written proof of the town's Soviet history had largely vanished. It is this apparent disconnect and absence of written documents that prompted me to use the label "(pre-)history" in this section's heading. However, this "prehistoric" Soviet past cast a heavy shadow on how residents engaged with the present, and it also channeled and directed hopes for the future. As we saw, the ghost of the Soviet past had come to life even in documents of a "city" administration that was administering a "settlement of urban type."

Destabilized World

> You should have come here ten years ago! Do you see this bank note? [I am being shown a bank note that is perfectly folded into the shape of a shirt.] These ten rubles used to be enough to buy a man's shirt! Our shops were the best in the region. They always had meat and fish, and sometimes even Dutch cheese! You know, back then we had Moscow provisioning [*moskovskoe obespechenie*]. Now we have nothing.
>
> KYRGYZ man, former miner, in his forties

When there was the Soviet Union our city was prestigious. We lived proudly;
we had Moscow provisioning. We didn't worry about tomorrow. We had
everything. Health care and education were for free. On Sundays we would
rest in the city park. We were all equally rich, and happy. But now, when we
go out it is like stepping into a nightmare.

KYRGYZ woman, teacher, in her fifties

These voices from the second half of the 1990s were typical of the immediate post-Soviet period, when comparisons with the Soviet past were on
everyone's mind. The most frequently invoked term in such comparisons
was "Moscow provisioning." Literally, this referred to the privilege enjoyed by industrial towns of strategic significance to be directly provided
with consumer goods from Moscow, instead of having to rely on slower,
longer, and leaner distribution channels that passed through two retail divisions, republican (SSR) and provincial (*oblast*). In practical terms this
meant that the state shops in Kokjangak had a greater variety of food than
those elsewhere, and that consumer goods ranging from shoes to furniture
were more frequently available. Town dwellers were envied for this privilege, and would often act as brokers to secure scarce goods for relatives in
less privileged places.

It might seem odd that this Moscow provisioning occupied such a central place in the collective memory given that after 1991 consumer goods
became much more widely available. The significance of Moscow provisioning, however, was that it highlighted two valued aspects of Soviet life,
and in so doing also symbolized the post-Soviet downfall. The first is that
during Soviet times, the goods and services that were available had always
been affordable. In fact, well-paid workers such as miners and engineers
were often unable to spend their entire earnings, because housing, transportation, and basic food items were subsidized and available at little cost,
while luxury items were hard to come by. This situation was reversed in
the 1990s when affordability instead of availability became the primary
concern. The reference to Moscow provisioning was thus also a critique of
a situation in which goods and services had become more expensive and
prices less predictable, a period in which living standards had plunged.
Second, apart from strictly economic concerns Moscow provisioning in-
dexed a "cultural and aesthetic connection—of the 'center in the periph-
ery,'" as Reeves (2014a, 114) has helpfully suggested. To receive Moscow
provisioning was an indicator of significance and privilege within the

Soviet political economy. It conjured a sense of modernity, of being cultured, educated, and Russophone, and in doing so it produced a sense of distinction from, and superiority over, other settlements in the region. As will be shown below, the loss of this privileged position contributed to a sense of existential and epistemological anxiety.

* * *

> After finishing education, you were expected to arrange your employment within a few months. If not, the police would call on your house. . . . It turns out that back then we lived well but didn't want to work, whereas now there is no one who forces us to work, and we end up sitting at home, which turns out to be very bad. (Nurbek, Kyrgyz man in his late forties)

Surely not everyone cherished memories of police checks on slackers, but the underlying positive valuation of order was a common theme. When we talked, in 2008, the memory of compulsory work must have looked particularly attractive to Nurbek, because apart from infrequent casual work as a driver he had indeed been "sitting at home" for several years, in sharp contrast to the stable employment and sufficient income he had enjoyed during the first ten years of his adult life. Unemployed and in his late forties, in 2008 he was living with his two teenage children, dependent on remittances sent by his wife, who was working in the Russian city of Novosibirsk and had not been home in eighteen months.

During Soviet times, Kokjangakians largely relied on salaried income (more so than collective farmers in the neighboring villages, who had private plots and livestock) and were thus greatly affected by the loss of coal-mine and factory jobs. Diversifying the income base was difficult because the possibilities for animal husbandry and cultivating crops were limited in this urban environment. Households initially resorted to reductive strategies (saving on food) as well as depleting strategies, which involved the selling of furniture and other household items. The most common regenerative activities during this period were petty trading and circular migration, but these activities often failed to generate sufficient profit and sometimes even resulted in further indebtedness (Howell 1996, 68–70). Access to state benefits became more important from the mid-1990s onward, but the amounts would cover only a small part of household needs. The selling of construction materials from abandoned houses and other buildings was an important regenerative activity for as long as it lasted (roughly 1995 to 2005). Small-scale mining started to develop when the coal mine was closed entirely in 1999. Increasingly, remittances sent by a spouse or child working abroad (usually in Russia) were critical to many households.

What the new sources of income had in common was that they were unpredictable in terms of availability and reward, in stark contrast to bureaucratically organized Soviet industrial labor. The case of coal mining is instructive. Nurbek often emphasized the "order" (*poriadok*) of work in the mine. Work back then had been tough but also honest (*chestnaia*), with its ten-hour shifts, regular payments, and prospect of early retirement. He shared stories about the family feel of his work party (*komanda*), his "stern but just foreman" who he had admired as a young man, about the expertise of specialists who were responsible for planning and safety, and the authority of the (Russian) director. This bureaucratic and patrimonial structure had caused its own frictions, but nevertheless stood in marked contrast to the informal mining activities that had come in its stead.[9] The men involved in these new small-scale mining activities rarely had access to air drills or other power equipment, instead using crowbars, pickaxes, and shovels to dig mine shafts into the hills, often working for weeks underground without protection, and without knowing whether they would hit a coal layer.

* * *

During Soviet times, each neighborhood was different. The center and the Twenty-Third Quarter were mostly Russian, [Neighborhood] Forty was a mix of Uzbeks, Tatars, and others. The Kurds and Baptists each lived closely together [at the outskirts] as if in their own village. We would rarely go there; it felt strange. We Kyrgyz lived almost everywhere, but hardly in the center. Somehow that was considered to be too European. (Nurbek)

The sketched pattern suggests an ethnic mosaic rather than the kind of melting pot that Soviet texts proudly proclaimed when mentioning the number of nationalities coexisting and cooperating in its cities. The mix was diverse, but inhabitants tended to cluster together on the basis of origin, ethnicity, and religion. In everyday speech, the category "Russians" included Ukrainians but not the Russian Baptists, who were categorized separately on the basis of religious affiliation. The Kurds, who had been deported from the Georgian border region with Turkey to destinations across Central Asia in 1944, all lived together in a couple of streets, whereas Tatars lived interspersed throughout the town. Interethnic marriages were not exceptional. They were fairly common between Tatars and Russians, as well as between Tatar and Russian women and Kyrgyz men, but several of the other groups, such as Kurds, Baptists and Uzbeks, observed more strictly the norm to marry among "one's own."

Positive references to the former heterogeneity abounded and usually glossed over the coercive roots and persistent inequalities of the mix. Thus, when talking about some of the architectural highlights of the town, it was pointed out that they reflected the skills of their German constructors, without mentioning that these Germans had been prisoners of war working in forced-labor projects. And when discussing the rapid expansion of town, it was rarely mentioned that this was achieved in no small measure through the forced labor of deported groups from the Caucasus. Others spoke approvingly of the many "cultured" (*kulturnye*) and "learned" (*uchennye*) Russians who occupied the top ranks of the mine and factory management, without reflecting on the inequalities between "Europeans" and "Asians" in the Soviet economy. But whatever the imperfections and underlying tensions of the Soviet internationalist ideal, the diversity of the population was remembered positively as having made Kokjangak a "real" (*nastoiashchii*) city, and one that was "cultured."

The exodus of the 1990s not only sliced the population in half but also radically altered its composition. Whereas up to 1990 Russians and other "Europeans" made up approximately 50 percent of the population, this dropped to a mere 9 percent by 2004 when 75 percent of its population was ethnically Kyrgyz.[10] The first to leave had been those with good prospects for resettling elsewhere, among whom the vast majority of residents with professional and family connections in Russia and Ukraine.[11] Notwithstanding the overwhelming out-migration, the town saw a few newcomers as well, mostly recently divorced women who came to Kokjangak because apartments could be bought at prices close to zero. Although the size of the population stabilized in the mid-1990s at around ten thousand, this was only a deceptive stability, with many remaining residents using Kokjangak as a resting point in their increasingly migratory lives.

In short, Kokjangak's population became much more homogeneous in terms of ethnic and educational indicators, and in the process became increasingly similar to neighboring rural settlements. Possibly because of this flattening, some inhabitants became even more inclined to stress the distinctiveness of urban life. Thus, the town's Kyrgyz inhabitants often prided themselves on having a better command of Russian than Kyrgyz people living elsewhere, and many Kyrgyz parents tried to get their children placed in the one remaining Russian-language school.[12] When in 2010 conflicts erupted between Kyrgyz and Uzbeks in the nearby city of Jalalabad and in several smaller settlements in the region, my Kyrgyz acquaintances told me that such violence would not happen in Kokjangak because its inhabitants were more "civilized" (*tsivilizovannye*). It had, after all, been a mining town.[13] This urban legacy was particularly treasured by the older generations, those who had invested most in the Soviet ideal of modernity. But despite their best efforts, the downfall of the town was unstoppable, and outsiders had come to associate Kokjangak with poverty, crime, and disease.

*   *   *

These |five-story apartment buildings| used to be the most prestigious living quarters—they had all the amenities |*udobstvie*|. They are no longer prestigious, of course. About half the apartments are empty. Did you hear this joke about "going to the fifth floor"? . . . No? Well, it is better that way |Nurbek says with a knowing smile|.[14]

The amenities in these centrally located apartments (built in the 1970s) were running water, central heating, electricity, gas, and built-in kitchens and bathrooms with plumbing. That is, they had the amenities that were lacking in most freestanding houses and older apartment buildings (such as the *barak* and the *kommunalka*). The first tenants of these apartments belonged to the privileged layers of society; they were employed in managerial and engineering positions, or had good jobs in the city administration. However, none of these positive connotations still held. The roofs had started to leak, the central heating and gas had long been disconnected, and water had to be carried with buckets to the top floors because of low water pressure in the pipes. Moreover, former occupants had often stripped their apartments of window seals, doors, and floors on departure, leaving gaping

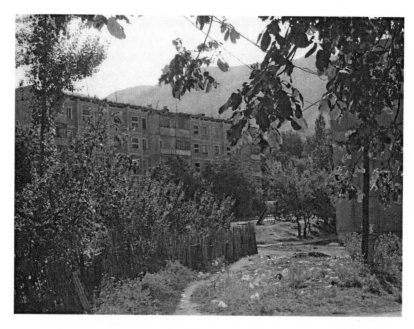

The five-story apartment buildings in the center of Kokjangak, August 2009

holes in the buildings. A clear indicator of decline was that in 2004 apartments were sold for as little as forty dollars.[15] The city center was not only being emptied out in a material sense, it also became perceived as a black hole in moral terms, as already suggested by Nurbek's comment above. Single mothers occupied the least desirable top floors, and residents of all floors were those with few other options, among whom were many elderly Russians. It had become a place of last resort, known for its frequent scandals related to domestic and other violence, drug abuse, and alcoholism.

In the center of town it was not just the high-rises that were collapsing; most freestanding houses were vanishing altogether. These houses were bought up by middlemen who were primarily interested in the construction materials, leaving nothing behind but the concrete foundations. But while the formerly prestigious city center was emptied out, the outlying neighborhoods experienced a different dynamic. These had been less prestigious because of their distance from shops and workplaces as well as their lack of amenities. But given the collapse of urban infrastructure, such considerations had lost their relevance, while at the same time the advantages of living in the outskirts had grown in significance: the larger backyards allowed for cultivating vegetables, growing fruit, and keeping some cattle, while their location provided better access to pastureland. Certainly, the outlying neighborhoods also lost a significant part of their population, but many of the abandoned houses (including a few two-story apartment buildings) were being reused as stables or storage places. Kadyr, for example, had gone to some length to register his neighbor's property under his own name. He then transformed the neighboring house into a stable for raising bulls and for storing hay and wood, and merged the two yards into a sizable vegetable plot.

The result of these processes is a town with a hole in the middle—a couple of largely empty administration buildings in the midst of ruins and decaying apartment buildings—with life continuing in the increasingly village-like neighborhoods. This centrifugal dynamic was not contained within city boundaries; the loss of city status and reclassification as "settlement of urban type" meant that residents were now required to travel to the district (*raion*) capital (thirty-five kilometers to the south) for many administrative issues. Moreover, as mentioned, residents increasingly depended on "the beyond" for work and for remittances. In the 2000s most families had one or several members who were engaged in ongoing circular migration to Russia, in particular to Ekaterinburg and Novosibirsk.[16] Inhabitants felt that while in previous times they had been living in a place that mattered, they had ended up on the margins of even their own networks. No longer the pinnacle of Soviet modernization it had been in the past, Kokjangak started to blend in with the rest of the region.

To recapitulate, the memory of Moscow provisioning was so powerful because it gave voice to the experience of deprivation in the present: the disappearance of Soviet industry and its supporting economy; a demographic transition that signified severance from the centers of power; and a spatial inversion that indicated the town's growing irrelevance and moral downfall. Life in Kokjangak had not only become bleak in purely economic terms; the pain was intensified by a sense of disorientation, and the loss of relevance and status.

What was lost in the midst of economic hardship was a sense of being distinctively modern, with "modern" here referring to the idea of being

advanced (in comparison to the past and in comparison to neighboring locali-
ties) as measured by education, technology, and consumption. These indicators had always been celebrated in official descriptions of the city and summed
up in statistics detailing the metric tons of excavated coal, the number of hospital beds, the kilometers of paved roads, the capacity of the stadium, and the
number of yearly visits to the cinema. This emphasis on numbers had produced a "quantified modernity" that functioned to smooth over the problems
of the Soviet project. The strategy never succeeded entirely, and inhabitants
had been painfully aware of the shortcomings of the Soviet modernist project
and the coercion and contradiction on which it was built. Nevertheless, this
quantitative surface had provided a semblance of modernity that continued
to provide a compelling frame of reference. Moreover, this quantified modernity, with its always-increasing numbers, had been explicitly future oriented. As a "work-in-progress" (Hirsch 1997), as a past imperfect in which
there was relative stability and hope of a better future, the Soviet project continued to nourish longing thoughts long after its decay.

This forward-looking Soviet "work-in-progress" was experienced as
not only having come to a standstill but of moving in reverse. The references to a better past, of a city that had been modern and cosmopolitan,
suggested a process of decline, as also seen in the use of descriptors of the
present such as "primitive," "loss," and "dying city." Moreover, inhabitants experienced the new situation as one of chaos in which the stability
and predictability of the late Soviet period had given way to uncontrollable
flux. In order to highlight this aspect of uncontrollability, it might be appropriate to refer to the changes not as a process of "demodernization" but
as a process of becoming "postmodern." In a short but insightful article,
Unni Wikan (1996) presents the life story of a Buddhist nun in Bhutan,
whose experiences with abuse, death, and oppression Wikan interprets as
"an extreme example of a typical condition of things falling apart," and
suggests that this can be taken "as a prototype for postmodern life" when
approached from the perspective of the dispossessed (1996, 279). In Kokjangak residents had been forced out of the relative comfort zone that their
island of Moscow provisioning had provided. The world no longer came to
their city, and so its inhabitants were forced to go out to the world, becoming in the process more cosmopolitan than they previously had been.

This tilting of perspective is not to dismiss or downplay the effects of
impoverishment and dispossession but to acknowledge the flip side of this

process. In the words of Caroline Humphrey, "The dispossessed are people who have been deprived of property, work, and entitlements, but we can also understand them as people who are themselves no longer possessed" (2002, 21). Or, as Magnus Marsden shows, despite cosmopolitanism often being associated with affluent urbanites, conditions of marginalization and uncertainty may just as well foster an attitude of open-endedness, thereby enhancing "potentialities for engagements with others" (2008). But before moving to a discussion of the ways that inhabitants of Kokjangak held on to lost values and reached out to new ideas, let's first explore in more detail how inhabitants navigated this uncertain terrain.

Navigating Post-Soviet Chaos

The closure of the coal mine had allowed the big shots to enrich themselves and had pushed ordinary people into poverty. That much was certain, but the reasons for closure and the techniques of enrichment were hotly debated and contested in the late 1990s, and into the early 2000s.

There were those who argued that the coal mine had had its days; the increasing length of the shafts indicated that the coal reserve was almost depleted and that coal mining had stopped making economic sense even in the last years of the USSR. "The thing is," a former engineer told me, "metal and wood [for scaffolding] are expensive and coal is cheap, so when the coal is too deep it no longer makes sense." The investments required for scaffolding, ventilation, and excavation had started to outweigh the value of the extracted coal, which led to collapse as soon as the planned economy was replaced with a market economy in which prices of commodities were no longer fixed at politically convenient levels by the central government. But there were others who argued that closure had been due to a tragic policy mistake. In the mid-1990s the Akaev government decided the country would switch from a coal-based energy supply to one based on hydroelectric energy, oil, and gas. The decision backfired when price levels of imported oil and gas quadrupled, and nationally produced hydroelectric power proved unable to meet demand. Undoing the mistake was complicated because by that point the coal mines had already deteriorated and required massive investments. In the case of Kokjangak such investment was not forthcoming, and several potential investors had withdrawn after having expressed initial interest. Finally, and this was the most widespread opinion, there were those who said that it had all been intentional; directors and politicians had conspired in order to benefit from the bankruptcy and subsequent privatization.

Whether closure had been inevitable, a tragic mistake, or the result of conspiracy, it allowed successive directors—there had been four between 1991 and closure in 1999—to enrich themselves. The largest misappropriation took place in the early 1990s when the director and his associates, together with officials from Bishkek, pocketed a series of grants originally intended to secure the mine's future. Next, while the mine's scale of operation was being downsized, its inventory started disappearing. There was a persistent rumor about what happened to the relatively new and very expensive excavators (that had been purchased in the late 1980s). The official line was that they were irretrievable—buried inside a deep mine shaft following a gas explosion—but several insiders insisted that the explosion happened after the excavators had been removed, and only happened so as to cover up the stealthy sale of this equipment to buyers from China. Verifying such stories was complicated by the fact that each of the four directors left Kokjangak as soon as a successor appeared on the scene. Moreover, any paper trail—if it had ever existed—disappeared with the closure of the mine in 1999.

The exact history of accumulation and dispossession remains, and most likely will remain, unknown. In fact, if this history could have been documented in detail, it would never have taken place. The techniques of enrichment existed only because they were shrouded in a haze, the details remaining undocumented and knowable only by proxy. This fogginess was characteristic not just of the mine but more generally of the political-economic space that inhabitants navigated.[17] As we will see, the condition of uncertainty had implications that pointed beyond the economic to ethical, epistemological, and ontological concerns.

* * *

Almaz was visibly annoyed: "Right when we finally reached the coal the officials [*chinovniki*] appeared, demanding their share. They haven't given us a thing—no salary, no equipment, nothing. That is how things are here. They neither provide work, nor do they allow us to work." We had a shot of vodka and the conversation switched to more frivolous matters, but the issue must have continued to occupy his mind, because not much later Almaz added, "Actually we are helping lots of people. Some people plant grain, others tomatoes, and we dig coal. People need coal. That is how it should be, right? But our officials, they don't care, they come when they want to fill their pockets. But when we need them, they say: 'We won't give you anything.'"[18] A honking car arrived, and after quickly buying two more bottles of vodka, Almaz took his leave to join his friends, while I remained behind with Lola in her kiosk. "These guys don't earn that poorly. Actually they are my best clients," Lola commented. "But I wouldn't want to be in their place, going into those holes not knowing if you will ever see daylight again."

When I first got to know Almaz, in early 2004, he was nineteen years old and was in between things, quite literally. He officially lived with his parents but in practice spent most nights at one of his friends'. He somewhat studied for a bookkeeping degree as an external (*zaochnyi*) student, the main activity for which, he told me, consisted of making the right payments. In any case, he did not think a degree would land him a job, it was just that his parents insisted he should have one. Since his final year in school (two years previously) he had been working off and on in small-scale mining as an *apache*. The name *apache* was used for the (mostly young) men who were engaged in the most informal of mining activities, and was based on similitude. In the words of an acquaintance, "It is because they run in the mountains like the Apaches, just as we know it from the movies." Finding the coal layers was a laborious process of trial and error. With the aid of only shovels and picks, Almaz and his mates would dig narrow shafts into the mountain slope in search of coal, usually between ten and twenty meters deep before hoping to hit a thin layer of coal (eighty centimeters thick). Several times Almaz's group had worked in vain for weeks.

Over the following months Almaz continued to work as an *apache*, but his attitude seemed to be changing. We talked a week after a tragic incident happened at a short distance from where he had been working. A young guy had been inside a shaft when it collapsed. He was dead by the time his mates managed to dig him out. Several men died from such accidents each year, but according to Almaz, "no one really knows because people don't want to talk about it." One reason for this silence was that public attention could very well bring an end to informal mining, thereby shutting off the main source of income for many families.[19] This particular tragedy had gotten under Almaz's skin. Even though he rationalized the tragedy by saying that those guys had been working in a dangerous spot—a week earlier their shaft had partly caved in after rainfall—seeing this happen at such proximity made the risks of these kinds of mining activities very palpable. "When you are inside the mine it is OK, you just work like mad," he said. "But waking up in the morning knowing that you have to go back in, that's the worst."

Almaz had been making plans to find work in Russia. In 2005 he traveled to Ekaterinburg in Russia, where he joined a group of Kyrgyz men from Kokjangak in construction. For the next three years we were out of contact, but when I returned to Kokjangak in 2008, Almaz was there as well, once again engaged in mining activities. He had worked in Russia for a year and a half, but preferred not to talk about his experiences, which had brought him very little of value, including financially: "You know, work in the mines is dangerous, but what are the alternatives? Our people also die in Russia." Possibly his negative experiences in cold, faraway Russia had made him more accepting of the dangers of mining at home. But something else had changed as well. Almaz had started to become interested in Islam.

When I visited Almaz at his workplace in 2008, he introduced me to his foreman, who was also an active member of the conservative Islamic movement Tablighi Jamaat (see also chapter 4). We had a short conversation in which I asked him about his views on the dangers of mining and the troubles caused by the *chinovniki*. I did not manage to record a verbatim script of his words, but they were close to the following: "Look, in here we trust in Allah; the future cannot be known; we are earning money; we are able to provide for our families; Allah is really great." Later, Almaz told me that his new work group (*komanda*) was very different from what he had experienced before: the men were all serious and supportive, and they had a responsible leader. Moreover, his own life had changed. No longer did he spend his earnings on alcohol, but instead he was making plans for marriage. Whether due to his experiences in Russia, his involvement with Islam, or both, Almaz came across as more mature and self-confident.

As all young people in Kokjangak, Almaz found himself confronted with numerous uncertainties and dangers, needing to navigate an environment in which there were no good alternatives, only least bad options. Almaz's complaints about the *chinovniki* at the beginning of this section had contained important hints for how to understand the post-Soviet condition. His statement about honest labor—"that is how it should be, right?"—suggested that he neither opposed "planned economy" nor "the free market" per se, but rather resented the decay of the former and the impotency of the latter, which had resulted in a "wild market." The *chinovniki* were exemplary of this: they had been a necessary evil of the bureaucratic Soviet system, who in the new conditions had turned into parasitic predators backed by fake documents and a corrupt legal system. The sense of chaos was precisely this, not the absence of order—a free-for-all—but rather the unfairness and unreliability of the remnants of Soviet bureaucracy. In the midst of this chaos Almaz had been in search of justice and stability, which in 2008 he found not in the state or an economic ideology, but in the authority of an informal religious leader.

* * *

Lola had been charged with drug possession and spent three nights in jail, losing 20,000 Kyrgyz som (KGS) |which amounts to 400 USD] on her way to the judge. Eventually her case was dropped, but she still had to come up with an additional 5,000 KGS to cover procedural expenses, or they would reverse the process and put her on trial anyway. When I asked if these were legal payments she answered: "I don't know, but they told me that it was according to the law and they showed me a document. Now I have to find 5,000 som. At home they scold me because of all these extra expenses." Atyrgul commented dismissively that it was never about the law but about how much money they could squeeze out of Lola, and added: "If I would be president, everything would be different." We all laughed.

Atyrgul was intimately familiar with these problems. In fact, her brother had been imprisoned just a few months previously, and was about to be transferred to a prison in the north of the country. The charges were drug possession and use of violence. Atyrgul acknowledged that her brother was sometimes involved in shady business, but she didn't believe that to be the reason for his imprisonment, speculating that the police officers had planted the drugs on him. "I know these police officers. This is how they make money. They put someone in prison, wait for relatives to buy him out, and split the money." Atyrgul herself had collected money from friends and relatives to buy her brother out of jail, but the required bribes turned out to be too high in his case. She had come back frustrated: "There is no good police, they are like mafia. The judges are the same. It doesn't matter who the [accused] is, they will assume he is guilty. They only listen to the police."

Three years previously, after she and her "good-for-nothing" husband separated, Atyrgul had moved to a fifth-floor apartment with her two children. She was not someone to complain, but confided that having to be "husband and wife at the same time" drove her to despair at times. When we talked in May 2004 she had held her job at the military office for about a year. She had found the job through an acquaintance, and in order to actually be appointed she only had to "throw in" (*kidat'*) the modest amount of 500 KGS (10 USD), plus a month of work without pay. Her main task was to contact the families whose sons were being drafted into the military. When she told me that her monthly salary was 1,050 KGS, an amount vastly insufficient to feed a family of three, I asked her: "But how do you actually live?" She replied: "I don't know . . . well, sometimes I'm lucky at work."

The following week I accompanied Atyrgul on one of her routes, contacting families with sons soon to be enlisted. At one point I waited on the street while Atyrgul was conversing with a woman inside a courtyard, and when she returned she reported that the woman had asked her to make inquiries at the military office in Suzak (the district center), and given her 500 KGS for this purpose, hoping that she would manage to return with the *voennyi bilet* (literally, "war ticket," which provides deferral or exemption from being drafted). "Being lucky" meant running into a family that was prepared to go to some length to keep their son out of the army. In most cases she received only a small fee for assisting in getting a deferral, but some families aimed at removing their sons from the register altogether, a more complicated and lucrative procedure. "It's not huge money," Atyrgul explained, "my boss gets fifty and I get fifty [USD]."

Later that day, the town-hall cashier refused to release Atyrgul's salary because her boss (in Suzak) had not been coming to work for over two weeks and thus had not signed off on her paycheck. Atyrgul made a scene, phone calls were made, and she was promised that her paycheck would be available for collection the following day. She commented to me that she hoped her boss would be made redundant, which would give her a chance to get his job instead. Sure, she would have to hand money to the army officer (*polkovnik*) in Suzak, but she was optimistic that she would be able to collect the amount needed. Atyrgul always talked matter-of-factly about these realities, thereby indicating that harboring any (Weberian-style) ideal-type notions of bureaucracy would be entirely out of place. She navigated this messy reality by presenting herself as a strongheaded woman, a fighter (*boevaia zhenshchina*) not afraid of anyone. The arrest of her brother, as much as it affected Atyrgul negatively, had at least the mildly positive effect of strengthening her tough image, as someone from a scandalous family (*skandal'naia sem'ia*) who was not to be messed with.

Atyrgyl actively worked the tensions between corrosive bureaucratic structures and flexible informal arrangements. As a skilled and self-conscious actor she managed to survive, making small sums of informal money every once in a while. But ultimately this "chaotic" system worked against people like her, against those who lived on the margins of society and were unable to mobilize strong support networks. In fact, when I tried to get in touch with her in 2009 I failed. Lola told me that Atyrgyl had lost her job the year before, and had taken her two children to Bishkek in search of work and a better future.

* * *

Lola and her friends Chinara and Atyrgul were discussing the local Peace Corps Volunteers. Lola suggested that they were spies, but Chinara interjected: "What spies? There is nothing here that can be of interest to their government." Atyrgul replied that she had heard that the volunteers were sent over by the US government as a form of punishment, because why else would someone come to Kokjangak? Without reaching consensus, Chinara concluded: "Anyway, they have their own businesses. Take Carrie, she made a deal with Khatamov [director of the town's employment center], and together they split the money. Did she ever contribute to some kind of [community] project, or give people money? No, of course not, she kept the money herself." Atyrgul half jokingly said that this showed how well Carrie had adjusted to Kyrgyz reality, and it prompted her to mention the Kyrgyz saying: "If you fail to eat the meat of others like a wolf, your own meat will be taken" (Karyshkyr bolup biröönün, etim zhulup albasam, senikin zhulup alat).

The lack of trust, the sense of suspicion, and the notion that everyone becomes drawn into this "post-Soviet chaos" was evident in this conversation. The reference to wolves' dinner etiquette reflected the idea that life in Kokjangak amounted to a zero-sum struggle, and brought to mind Hobbes's state of nature in which "the condition of man . . . is a condition of war of everyone against everyone." In fact, the same human-animal comparison featured in the Greek saying from which Hobbes had taken his inspiration: "*homo homini lupus est*" (a man is a wolf to another man).[20] Just like in Hobbes, the reference to animalistic behavior contained a negative value judgment, suggesting that order is to be preferred over chaos, a sentiment we also came across in the various nostalgic references to the Soviet past. The post-Soviet condition, in the words of my acquaintances, was to be seen as *dikii* (untamed) or as *bardak* (chaos), a term with the secondary meaning of "brothel," thus weaving ideas of moral decay into discussions of animal-like struggle.

Notwithstanding the similarities, my acquaintances' descriptions of "post-Soviet chaos" reveal important differences with the Hobbesian state of nature. Inhabitants of Kokjangak did not suggest that chaos followed from the equality of citizens in the absence of a "power able to over-awe them all" (Hobbes 1651). Instead of pure randomness, what was sketched was a situation in which hidden orders loomed below a seemingly orderless surface. Here, just like in chaos theory, chaos referred not to pure disorder but to "order within apparent disorder," possibly even to "deterministic kinds of order . . . arising from the generalized properties of complex dynamical systems" (Mosko 2005, 7). The miners argued that the main problem was not the collapse of the state but the remainders thereof; the women insisted that the police had turned into a predatory machine targeting ordinary people, and they suggested that local NGO representatives plotted to channel external funds into their own pockets.

The logics underlying these observed predatory practices were tacitly understood, and the tactics employed were recognized by all. However, the efficacy of these practices depended on remaining in the shadow of the largely empty rhetoric of privatization, bureaucracy, and development. Moreover, precisely because of their shadowy nature these tactics were never hegemonic.[21] In other words, the overwhelming sense of chaos and unpredictability was not caused by random disorder, but because informal hierarchies, networks, and lines of exclusion operated below the surface.

Not only did these hidden orders cause uncertainty, they produced and enlarged inequalities in ways that were difficult to predict.

The ethnographic examples in this chapter all reveal aspects of this chaotic configuration. The collapse of the Soviet infrastructure had produced a rush for spoils that inhabitants presented as chaotic, in which the activities of the police, officials, NGO workers, and Peace Corps Volunteers were characterized by secrecy and obscurity. Far from being "random," everyone recognized the logics of dependency, reciprocity, and protection on which they were based. The rush for spoils had the "predictable" effect of enriching the well-placed and leaving poorly connected inhabitants increasingly impoverished and marginalized.

Chaos, then, is about the cracks through which people fall; it is about the opportunities it creates for those able to manipulate the situation and the immoral behaviors that people are pushed into. Ultimately, it is about the reordering of society at a moment when connections are unstable, in which new lines of inclusion and exclusions are being drawn and old ones are being reinstated or intensified. In such circumstances, Katherine Verdery comments, "people of all kinds could no longer count on their previous grasp of how the world works" and "became open to reconsidering . . . their social relations and their worlds of meaning" (1999, 35). Or, to go back to an already-mentioned observation by Geertz, "it is a loss of orientation that most directly gives rise to ideological activity" (1973, 219). It is to such reconsiderations and reorientations that we now turn.

Reorientation

On a cold morning in November 1998 a white UNDP jeep arrived in Kokjangak, coming to a halt next to a small office building. Two days previously a UNDP worker had made a phone call to a local NGO, expressing the intent to include the town in a "Participatory Poverty Alleviation Project," and therefore wishing to meet with poor inhabitants.[22] The phone call had not been without effect. A crowd of two hundred people had assembled in the open area in front of the NGO's office. The two UNDP workers, one of whom was me, struggled to get through the crowd into the office, which was equally packed. People were jostling to enter their names and passport data on long lists. As my colleague and I found out later, rumors had circulated that the UNDP was about to embark on a massive aid program. And instead of relying on local intermediaries—who, as everyone knew, would channel funds to their own people—this time the

UNDP would be working directly with recipients. Together my colleague
and I addressed the crowd outside while standing on top of the stairs leading
to the office. We explained that the project would not be handing out grants,
but would provide access to microcredit to poor residents after they had first
received various forms of training and been "socially mobilized" for at least
half a year. This had the desired effect of thinning out the crowd—those
who had expected immediate assistance left the scene—but at least a hundred
inhabitants stayed and came to subsequent meetings.

For a brief moment, the UNDP workers had produced a wave of anticipation in Kokjangak. Unavoidably, this initial enthusiasm slumped when
it became clear that no quick salvation was forthcoming. Nevertheless, in
the following weeks sixty inhabitants joined the Poverty Alleviation Program, which continued to run in Kokjangak for the next twelve years (and
would include up to two hundred inhabitants). When in 2008 I talked
again with some of the earliest participants about their experiences, several
mentioned the mix of anticipation and skepticism with which they had approached the project and its missionaries, only gradually becoming committed as the project got on its feet, something that was accompanied by
an adjustment of expectations as the project established its routine functioning, which included monthly meetings, training sessions, provision of
access to microcredit, and the initiation of small infrastructural projects.
To my acquaintances, the involvement of foreigners had been simultaneously promising because of their external position (which would potentially disrupt the usual patterns of exclusion) and worrying because of their
naïveté (which made them easy targets for manipulation by those in powerful positions).

I present this example because it provides a glimpse of the volatile dynamics of hope in a destitute environment and the "attitude of
open-endedness" (Marsden 2008) that had emerged. There are many reasons why this development mission never instilled the kinds of conviction that some political and religious missions managed to produce (even
if only temporarily). And yet the events made me think about the similarities and differences between the ways in which secular and religious
projects travel, the variations in the fluctuations of affect, and how external ideological projects become entangled with local views and interests.
In previous decades "activists" had raised awareness of the truth of "scientific atheism" and more broadly of socialism. In the new millennium
development activists had taught inhabitants about rights, sustainability,

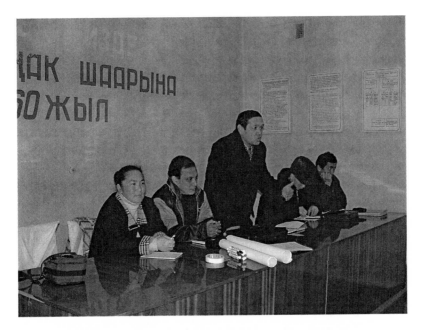

UNDP workers and their local counterparts holding a meeting in Kokjangak,
November 2003

and financial mechanisms; meanwhile Tablighi Muslim travelers tried to
impress on inhabitants the importance of coming closer to Islam; several
Pentecostal missions aimed at bringing the "Good News" of the New Tes-
tament; leaders of the opposition rallied inhabitants to join them in oust-
ing the government; and spiritual healers offered solutions tailored to the
problems of individuals. These multiple visions alternately focused on the
here and now or the afterlife, differently emphasized the collective or the
individual, and demanded a break with the past or instead tried to demonstrate continuity. As we will see in the next chapters, each of these characteristics influenced the specific rhythms, intensities, and reach of concrete
ideological currents.

At the start of this chapter I quoted a *Vechernii Bishkek* newspaper article stating that "it is not difficult to destroy a city. One does not even need
to bomb it. All that needs to be done is to take away hope and belief in
tomorrow. Then the city will destroy itself."[23] In some ways this had been
true enough—the city had indeed collapsed with the emigration of half its

population and the closure of the mine and the factories. Nevertheless, the materials contained in this chapter suggest that the relation between hope and destitution needs to be examined more closely, precisely because, as Zigon has titled an article, "Hope Dies Last" (2009). Even or especially in the direst of situations hope provides the "the energy, the petrol" needed to live and act. If we see hope as a method that reorients knowledge, directing it toward an imagined future (Miyazaki 2004), then the "taking away of hope"—the removal of one imagined future—will push people to imagine alternative ones. For many, this had meant a spatial relocation of hope: they had made the decision to leave the town, moving to horizons where they expected to have better lives. But even those who stayed behind found new points of reference in their "hopeless town."

Writing about the indigenous inhabitants of Sakhalin, Bruce Grant has made a related argument. He argues that in the twentieth century the Nivkhi were caught between two master narratives: a narrative of "cultural authenticity" that depicted the Nivkhi as "children of nature" with their own language, customs, and rituals; and a "stride" narrative that presented the Nivkhi as having leaped into modernity and become true modern Soviet citizens. But in the late 1980s, the modernist narrative imploded with the decline and collapse of the Soviet system, while the cultural authenticity narrative proved empty because much knowledge about "traditional" ways of living had vanished or was no longer relevant. However, Grant writes, they were "discovering symbolic capital amid the ruins of both these myths" (1995, 158).

How does the case of Kokjangak compare? More than anything else, the inhabitants of Soviet Kokjangak had identified with the modernist narrative. The memories of Moscow provisioning and the remainders of the modern Soviet mining city continued to influence people's expectations and desires. But with the state having lost its ability to project the future, having lost the "mechanisms for the projection of hope" (Hage 2003, 3), ideas of the modern started to connect in novel ways with tradition. Alexia Bloch argues that "the postsocialist condition requires us to pay close attention to competing ideologies and systems of meaning that give life to shifting subjectivities and the place of ideology in the multiple forms that modernity takes" (2005, 556). This is what I will do in the rest of the book, tracing a range of ideological movements and their spokespersons as they presented their vision and tried to convince residents of their truth. The chaotic nature of the post-Soviet condition rendered any new capital, whether economic, social, or symbolic, highly unstable. Nevertheless, these new ideologies pierce into this foggy future, even if only for a moment, as we will see in the chapters ahead.

Part II

Dynamics of Conviction

3

What Happened to Soviet Atheism?

It was July 2009, and after a day of various work activities, Kadyr and I drove up a hill overlooking Kokjangak, picked up some beers along the way, and sat in the grass, relaxing and talking about the things that were on our minds. Kadyr knew I had been asking people questions about atheism, and he decided to share the following anecdote, of which I had already heard other versions (and not only in Kyrgyzstan). The anecdote was about a young antireligious activist who had been sent to the summer pastures to lecture the herdsmen of the collective about evolution. When the activist finally finished his long and tedious lecture in which he had explained that our human ancestors were apes, one of the oldest herders raised his voice: "This is all very well, and I am willing to accept that *your* forefathers were apes, as long as it is clear that *mine* were decidedly human." We laughed, but it remained unclear what the laughter was about. Were we—or was Kadyr—simply laughing at the narrow-mindedness of the antireligious activist and the quick-wittedness of the herder? Or were we perhaps also ridiculing the old man as a remnant of an outdated worldview, as someone who could not be taken seriously either?

The anecdote and the ambivalence that spoke through it testify to the kinds of epistemological conundrums that Kadyr and many others of his generation and background experienced. Kadyr was in his late forties, married, with four children, living in a modest house on the outskirts of Kokjangak. He had studied in Bishkek (then still named Frunze), sub-sequently worked as an engineer in the coal mine, and, after the mine's closure, lived off his small plot of land and his modest income as direc-tor of a local credit union. Kadyr would describe himself as a Muslim, a designation that for him was tightly interwoven with Kyrgyz culture and tradition. If asked, he would add that he was "not close to religion," which referred to the fact that he never went to the mosque and did not pay attention to the pillars of Islam. His secular position resembled that of many middle-aged town dwellers and was linked to a set of values that reflected having lived through the late Soviet period. Though Kadyr had never cared about scientific atheism, and, as we saw, was happy to ridicule it, the larger Soviet framework to which atheism had been tied was still of relevance to how he saw himself: modern, educated, and cultured.

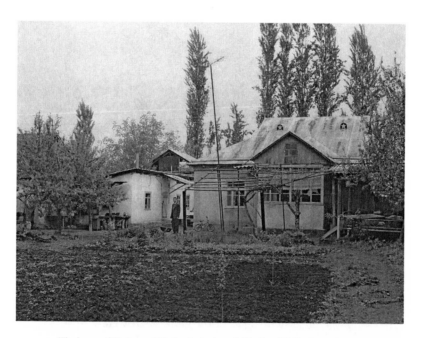

The home of Kadyr and his family in the neighborhood Kölmö, April 2004

In this chapter we will look at the ways in which people like Kadyr position themselves in relation to atheism, and subsequently gain insight into what happened to Soviet scientific atheism more generally. This atheism had vanished from public view in the early 1990s, almost as if its heavy-handed dissemination for a good seven decades had never taken place. As reflected in the anecdote, atheism came to be an object of ridicule and dismissal. In this chapter I ask what this public dismissal reveals not only about the "postatheist condition" but also about the features of "actually existing atheism" during the Soviet period. Drawing attention to contradictions in the architecture of atheism, I argue that the absence of a utopian dimension in Soviet atheism prevented its authentic realization and failed to incite lasting commitment and conviction in most people, which in turn enabled the swift removal of atheism at the end of the Soviet period.

However, the ambiguity of laughter suggested that the ridiculing and dismissal of atheism did not necessarily go very deep, and the anecdote could also be read as letting the antireligious activist off the hook. The staging of an elderly and presumably uneducated herder suggested apprehensiveness about religious ideas, in this case as a legacy of a "backward" past, but which was also linked to the idea that religiosity indicates narrow-mindedness. Such notions were particularly common among people who presented themselves as "not religious" or "not close to religion," whose anxieties were being fueled by the proliferation of new religious voices. In other words, the public dismissal of atheism did not mean that the various attitudes and ideas associated with it melted into thin air. Ironically, the public disappearance of atheism triggered renewed defenses of that which had never been desired.

Surface Disappearance

Back in 1999, when Soviet life was still a recent memory, I had a conversation with a friend who was an academic and former Communist Party member living in Bishkek, someone who referred to himself as being "not religious." The previous day he had watched, on his regular TV channel, a US-made documentary decrying evolutionary theory. The documentary had presented scientific evidence in support of the view that the world was only several thousand years old, and used this to uphold the strength of intelligent-design theory. "It is amazing," my friend told me, "all those years I had assumed that evolution was a fact, but, as it now turns out, that was just atheist propaganda." What interested me about this incident were not the specific strengths or weaknesses of either theory, but rather the reclassification of the "fact" of evolution into Soviet "propaganda" precisely because it happened in such an ad hoc manner. It suggested that because *all* previously acquired knowledge had potentially been propaganda (in the sense of having *deliberately* been distorted), knowledge itself had become unstable. But did this imply that atheism had simply evaporated? Or was the fact of evolution (and more broadly scientific atheism) perhaps never completely accepted as factual? And even if accepted as fact, what kind of intellectual and emotional investment, if any, did that indicate? For an investigation of these issues, a good point of entrance is the observation that evolutionary theory and atheist ideology vanished from the public sphere in August 1991. The contrast between two books from the early 1990s written by Kyrgyz scholars conveniently illustrates this disappearance of atheism from public discourse.

In 1991, before August of that memorable year,[1] Melis Abdyldaev, a Kyrgyz philosopher and scholar of atheism, published, in Russian, *Iz istorii religii i ateizma v Kyrgyzstane* (From the History of Religion and Atheism in Kyrgyzstan). The book contains a detailed history of the successes of the antireligious struggle, as well as the various obstacles that had to be overcome. His tone is often jubilant, and toward the end of the book he writes that "at present we have an entire battery of functioning people's universities of atheism" (1991, 110), delivering atheist activist graduates (*propogandisty–ateisty*) who are prolific in their activities. For example, one of Kyrgyzstan's provinces had no less than ninety teachers of atheism who gave a total of 2,221 lectures on atheism in the year 1986–87 (116–17). Abdyldaev acknowledges that the atheist project was by no means completed, and lists the familiar problems such as the use of crude and offensive techniques (109; see also Ro'i 1984, 31). But he envisions a bright future in which religion will have withered away, and he proposes that this goal will be reached faster if atheist activists engage more seriously with the philosophical basis of their project and proceed in nonconfronting manners, for example by promoting nonreligious rituals (1991, 126–27).

Just two years later, in 1993, another Kyrgyz scholar, Anara Tabysh-alieva, published (also in Russian) *Vera v Turkestane: Ocherk istorii religii Srednei Azii i Kazakhstana* (Belief in Turkestan: Essays on the History of Religion of Central Asia and Kazakhstan), which traces the history of various religious traditions. In a chapter titled "Soviet Times," Tabyshalieva mentions the closure of mosques and churches, the change of alphabet, the *hujum*, or unveiling campaigns, and the terror of the 1930s when believers were regarded as Trotskyites and imperialist spies (1993, 112–15), all as aspects of the long and erratic struggle against religion. But while Abdyl-daev focuses on the massive antireligious input, Tabyshalieva stresses the limited or even contradictory output. For example, she suggests that the cheap literature on atheism often functioned to trigger interest in religion (116),[2] and argues that the antireligious regime ultimately failed to inculcate atheist worldviews in its citizens. She concludes that "the renaissance of religiosity turned out to be the unexpected answer to the long and indifferent domination of atheism [and] the loss of belief in a communist or a socialist future" (122).

Tabyshalieva's book is an example of atheism's disappearance, of how it vanished almost overnight from scholarly work, political rhetoric, and public discourse. But at least the book still mentions Soviet atheism. Later texts on the history of religion published in Kyrgyzstan invariably reduced the Soviet atheist project to a couple of paragraphs at most, its authors often jumping from pre-Soviet to post-Soviet times (see, for example, Chotaeva 2004; Moldobaev 2002).[3] Political spokespersons equally distanced themselves from atheism, and used references to Muslimness and "nomadic spirituality," such as those found in the epic of Manas, to bolster their claims to power. It would be problematic to conclude from such trends that Kyrgyzstan was rapidly becoming a "religious place," but what is significant is that direct references to atheism had become conspicuously absent. The "atheist experiment" had become an object of ridicule, an awkward memory to be forgotten, and an increasingly irrelevant historical artifact.

When Tabyshalieva wrote that the renaissance of religion was the "unexpected answer," she touched on a core element in the argument that Alexei Yurchak later expounded in his book *Everything Was Forever, Until It Was No More* (2005). Writing about the Soviet system as a whole, he states that "although the system's collapse had been unimaginable before it began, it appeared unsurprising when it happened" (1). Yurchak solves this seeming paradox by arguing that the Soviet system and its ideology had been eroded from the inside out, and that people had already oriented themselves in new directions when the collapse occurred. Focusing on the role of language he documents the unfolding of a shift from "constative meaning" in which the content of ideological statements was understood to refer (relatively straightforwardly) to societal realities, to "performative meaning" in which ideological language becomes largely self-referential. In practical terms this meant that the content became subservient to the form, that is, both speakers and listeners increasingly focused on *how* things were being said, instead of *what* was being said. This "hegemony of form" obscured and destabilized the relation between signifier and signified, between ideological discourse and the reality to which it ostensibly referred.[4] Moreover, because the specific content of ideological language had become largely irrelevant, people became increasingly creative in looking for meaning elsewhere. In hindsight, this opened up creative possibilities that prepared Soviet citizens for the collapse, even if they had been unaware of it at the time.

Although Yurchak does not address atheism or antireligious discourse, the similarities are obvious. Scientific atheism had been an integral part of Soviet ideology, and Soviet citizens did not expect it to disappear before it actually did. Moreover, the hegemony of form had obscured the weaknesses of the antireligious efforts. This is not to say that the antireligious position was mere pretense. For teachers, atheist activists, and Communist Party members it constituted a discourse of familiarity and mutual understanding.[5] But even for them atheism did not in and of itself project an attractive vision onto the world. While people continued to *perform* allegiance to atheism, their attitudes had become increasingly ambivalent and ironic, so that once the Soviet Union collapsed, atheism could be dismissed without much further discussion.

Notwithstanding these similarities, the case of atheism has several distinctive features. Another reference to Tabyshalieva may clarify this. She speaks of the renaissance of religiosity as the answer to "the long and *indifferent* domination of atheism, to the social disruption and economic disappointments that were chaotically produced, and most importantly to the loss of *belief* in a communist or a socialist future" (1993, 122, emphasis added). Along with many authors Tabyshalieva writes about the disillusionment with the communist project that characterized the late Soviet period, but she appears to suggest, by using the word "indifference," that in the case of atheism the implicit *illusion* may never have existed. Hence the kinds of cynicism that ensued were of a different nature. Consider the well-known Soviet joke "They pretend to pay us and we pretend to work," which was popular precisely because it summed up the sense of disillusionment with the Soviet project and its disempowering effects. This joke could be easily translated to atheism, and many citizens of the Soviet Union would have agreed with the formulation "They pretend to eradicate religion, and we pretend to be atheists." But the effect is different. Whereas in the original anecdote everyone would agree on the importance of fair payment and the ultimate goals of (socialist) labor, in the reformulated version even the goal (of eradicating religion) was being questioned.

The important difference, then, seems to be that atheism never had a utopian element independent from the larger Soviet structure of which it was a part. This was evident when I asked an acquaintance if in her view atheism still existed, and received an answer full of surprise as to why I would even ask that question: "Atheism? All the institutions have disappeared!" At one level this was a straightforward truism, but what spoke through it was the assumption that "of course" the idea of atheism could never outlive its centralized institutionalized form.

Soviet atheism represented an extreme instance of the "hegemony of form" that had rendered ideological content redundant. This explains, to a degree, why Kyrgyz scholars, politicians, and ordinary citizens were able to distance themselves so quickly from the Soviet atheist project. There is a problem, though. If allegiance to atheism was largely about "form," can we not also postulate that atheism's dismissal was similarly about "form," giving us only very few insights into the continuities and discontinuities that operated below the surface? In other words, by answering one riddle—how and why did atheism disappear from public discourse?—we have created new ones. If we can speak of disappearance at all, what was it that had disappeared, and what had come in its stead?

The former communist mentioned in the beginning of this section had reclassified the "fact of evolution" as fantastic "propaganda," and had done so with relative ease because he had never been emotionally invested in this "fact." This calls for an exploration of what "actually existing atheism" had amounted to. Equally relevant to mention is the ad hoc nature of the former communist's reclassification. He was flirting with creationism at that very instance, but in later years would often talk dismissively about the new prominence of religious voices in the public and political domain. As will be documented below, atheism, to the extent that it existed, did leave important traces on people's attitudes and dispositions, which in spite of its surface disappearance would take on relevance in new contexts.

The Problem of Realizing Atheism

The suggestion "hegemony of form" provides an important clue for why atheism could be easily dismissed. But why did Soviet atheism fail to be emotionally and intellectually embodied? Yurchak's emphasis on the routinization of ideological language,[6] together with Weber's more encompassing argument regarding routinization through institutionalization (1968, 54–61), are important considerations, but these need to be augmented by an analysis of the architecture of atheist ideology itself. I provisionally hypothesize that an important reason for the "hegemony of form" in the case of atheism is that it is an empty ideology in the sense that it does not offer a forward-looking idea that allows people to identify with it or, in Althusser's words, to be interpellated by it.

Yurchak unwittingly points at the possibility of such a line of inquiry when he refers to Soviet ideology as a case of "failed interpellation" (2005, 116–17), but does so without following up on the brief reference to Althusser. Reconsider the anecdote of the atheist activist and the herdsman that started off this chapter. One of the many ironies of this anecdote is that, despite it having traveled widely across (post-)Soviet space, it is unlikely that such encounters happened often. The reason is that the failure of interpellation is a two-way process, as can be illustrated with reference to Althusser's original example, concerning the police officer who hails an individual—"hey, you there!"—at which the addressee turns round, and in the moment of turning becomes (is reaffirmed as) an ideological subject ([1971] 2008, 48).[7] The point of the comparison is not just that the herdsman who "turned" ridiculed and indeed emasculated the "police officer," but that the atheist activists were themselves often hesitant in hailing individuals. Instead of confidently hailing, they would hesitantly whisper, "Hey, you there." Frequently they would only "hail" on paper but not in person, or they would end up drinking vodka with the audience they were supposed to enlighten.

This may appear a flippant caricature, and we will have time to revisit it, but these are the elements that come through strongly in the complaints of late Soviet scholars. The problem with atheism in the 1970s and '80s was its inability to produce a compelling alternative to religion. Sure, the antireligious efforts did not lack in quantity (of publications, manpower, etc.), but they often lacked zeal. Thus, while the course Foundations of Scientific Atheism was being taught in hundreds of universities and technical high schools across the country, "complaints continued that there was much laxity and little enthusiasm on the part of students and instructors" (Pospielovsky 1987, 112). And while the "number of atheistic lectures . . . in Uzbekistan doubled from 28,289 in 1966 to 47,921 in 1976" (Kocaoglu 1984, 146), it was highly doubtful that these lectures (whatever number were actually delivered) convinced many people.

Notwithstanding the massive antireligious efforts (and not *only* on paper), Soviet sociologists acknowledged the lack of progress in inculcating atheist worldviews and attitudes. By 1981, writes Dimitry Pospielovsky, "the establishment's main concern was with the increasing amount of indifference to atheism and atheist propaganda, a kind of agnosticism as it were, in the ranks of the Soviet youth" (1987, 117). Some blamed this on the "conciliatory attitude to religion on the part of some communists and Komsomol members, and their participation in religious ceremonies and services" (Ro'i 1984, 33). Ro'i concludes on the basis of literature written by Soviet scholars in the Kyrgyz SSR that "atheistic propaganda lacked drive and specificity" (31). Working with similar literature David Powell concludes that "perhaps the most basic failure of atheist propaganda is its failure to reach believers" (1967, 372).

Atheism has a problem of interpellation because it lacks a utopian dimension or a "devotional core." Returning to Althusser, he argues that all ideology is centered around an "Absolute Subject" that "interpellates around it the infinity of individuals into subjects in a double mirror-connexion," thereby subjecting these individuals to itself "while giving them . . . the *guarantee* that this really concerns them and Him" ([1971] 2008, 54). But this understanding of ideology cannot be applied easily to atheism, as can be illustrated even by looking at the term itself. "Atheism" combines the prefix "a-" indicating "absence of," with the suffix

"-ism" indicating an active stance or ideology. That is, just like "amorality" indicates not immorality but the mere absence of morality, so can *a*-theism be seen as the mere absence of "theism" or religion. The more "active" or energized types of atheism can be either antagonistic or substantive. In the antagonistic version, atheism manifests itself as an *anti*-theism, deriving its fervor from its contrarian position. In the substantive version, atheism manifests itself as athe-*ism*, developing an alternative set of values to aspire to.[8] However, each of these possible versions of atheism contains an internal contradiction.

(Not) Remembering Soviet Atheism

As mentioned, in Kyrgyzstan after 1991, Soviet atheism had become an embarrassment of sorts, something preferably to be forgotten. Most people I spoke to simply dismissed the topic. This silence stood out precisely because other memories of the Soviet past were so readily communicated. My acquaintances in Kokjangak talked with pride about the heydays of their mining town, about the work ethic that had existed, and of having been part of a civilization in the making, just as they talked (with less enthusiasm) about the human sacrifices that had been made to produce this civilization and the corruption that accompanied its decay (see chapter 2). In contrast, people were highly reluctant to speak about atheism and antireligious efforts. When I would ask questions about it, the most typical response resembled the following one: "We just pretended to be atheists, but in our hearts we always believed [in God]." This response devalued atheism in the present, while the insistence on *pretense* suggested that Soviet atheism never had any value in the past either. Though this statement and similar ones confirm the failed interpellation of the previous section, it is important not to take them at face value. Pushing beyond people's knee-jerk reaction, I encouraged several former teachers and activists of atheism to elaborate on their views.

As a former school director, Asel' Kosobaeva was a respected inhabitant of Kokjangak. She had been schooled in scientific atheism but looked back at it with distaste. "Scientific atheism," she stressed, "is *such* a Soviet term, very vulgar [Russian, *vul'garnoe*] and coarse [*gruboe*], a simplistic distortion of religiosity." We spoke in her house, while her daughter-in-law brought in tea and food. She elaborated:

> Nowadays there is no one left who will say that they are atheist. But actually, we weren't atheists during the Soviet period either—back then we were also believers. Our God, the God of the Soviet people, was Marxism, Leninism, we were believers in the ideas of Marx and Lenin. And you see this [confirmed] when you go to the university [in Bishkek]. They have this Department of Religious Studies now, but its professors used to teach scientific atheism. That's absurd, isn't it?

Asel' rationalized her own involvement by saying, "Yes, I was a Komsomol member, an activist, a communist. That was all—how should I say it? . . . They didn't give us the possibility to think independently." Asked to give examples of the antireligious activism she used to be involved in, Asel' mentioned a trip with other activists to a village near Kokjangak:

> When we arrived in Oktiabr'skoe [village] we were directed to this Kyrgyz family, about whom [local teachers] were exasperated: "We have no idea what to do with them." The family turned out to be a young husband and wife, both in their twenties, Kyrgyz, who had become Baptists! So I asked them: "How can you be Baptists?! That is an *entirely* different faith! Are you not even thinking of your parents? This is a Muslim environment. It is fine that you are not Muslims, but you are Asians, so why . . . ?!" And then they answered. I didn't know what to say, so I just remained silent. They talked about their lack of basic means [of living]. Their parents had been poor: the husband's parents had died, the wife only had an elderly mother. And the Baptists had helped them, with money, with building a house. . . . You know, "Religion is the opium of the people." That's the basis, everything follows from that.

Asel's stories contain many interesting elements, ranging from the ways in which the relation between religion and culture was configured to the specifics of antireligious activism and the explicit suggestion about "opium of the people." Such leads will be followed up after we look at a few more viewpoints. What is worth emphasizing here is that during our conversation,

Asel' unreflectively shifted from a dismissal of atheism to a rejection of un-
orthodox forms of religiosity, such as in this case Russian Baptists, which
culminated in her affirmation of the "opium of the people" dictum.

Olga Nikolaevna, a Russian woman in her sixties, used to teach English in school number 1, the only school in Kokjangak still having a
Russian-language curriculum. After her two children moved away to
Bishkek and Russia, she and her husband thought about leaving as well,
but they considered themselves too old, and anyway, they both still had
work. She wasn't entirely sure why I wanted to talk about atheism:

> Atheism no longer exists, neither in the schools nor at the university. Those
> topics have disappeared, they are no longer propagated [*bol'she ne propagan-
> diruiut*]. On the contrary, nowadays it is religion that is propagated in the
> schools. In school number 4 the imam teaches "morality" from the Koran,
> and if more Russians had stayed in town, surely the Bible would have been
> used as well.

Olga told me that she had not thought about atheism in decades. "The thing
is," she added, "we learned scientific atheism so-so, just to pass the exam, and
that is why I don't remember much about it." She tried to find her old books
on atheism to refresh her memory for our conversation, but the books had
disappeared from the house. Although she had primarily taught English, she
also used to teach several "class hours" each week that were devoted to Soviet
citizenship. "We talked about the things that the plan stipulated: first was
patriotism; second was moral upbringing; third was religious and atheist education, and so on." When the focus was on atheist and antireligious topics
(once or twice a month), she prepared by reading popular literature and adjusting it to the age group she was teaching.

> For example, I would ask them: "One of the Ten Commandments is not
> to commit adultery—you really think that those priests stick to that rule?"
> That's how I tried to convince my pupils. . . . And I contrasted the childish
> primitiveness of religion with the flourishing of science in our country. For
> example, I would talk about the conquest of space [*kosmos*], asking the chil-
> dren: "If there was a God, surely the astronauts would have seen Him. But

did the astronauts see God? Is there at least one astronaut who did?" |Olga excused herself to go to the kitchen, and when she returned, she said:| I am surprised that I personally spoke those words in class. Now it turns out that some astronauts actually did see aliens, but that they were sent to mental institutions |*psikhushki*|. If they saw signs of an extraterrestrial civilization, they were too afraid to talk about it.

Olga's story is significant for a number of reasons, one of which is that it showed her past commitment to teaching, including teaching atheism, going to some length to translate and adjust the abstract message to her particular audience. This resonates with Sonja Luehrmann's observation about the effort and indeed sincerity of atheist teaching in the Autonomous Soviet Socialist Republic of Mari El, that through their engagement with atheist ideology, her informants fashioned themselves as Soviet teachers and practitioners (2011). While recollecting these memories Olga seemed almost surprised that she had held such strong views, a surprise that was probably related to her later flirtations with Orthodox and Pentecostal Christianity.

Svetlana Iussupovna used to be head of the Bishkek branch of the Knowledge Society (*Znanie*), the all-union society devoted to public lectures on scientific topics, and had been an active communist all her life.[9] Throughout our conversation she emphasized that the stories about the antireligious campaigns were all terribly exaggerated: "We never closed any churches or mosques, and we never imprisoned anyone because of his or her beliefs. Sure, I'm not denying that we fought [Russian, *borolis'*] against religion, but it was just a small part of everything else that we did. It came, maybe, on the tenth place." This was true even in a literal sense, such as when taking part in educational programs designed for pastoralists. "I was part of a campaigning team [*agitbrigada*], and when we traveled to the mountain pastures [Kyrgyz, *jailoo*], we would bring all kinds of things—about health, about agriculture, and also about atheism." She then continued to speak about the antireligious activities she had taken part in:

We never went to the mosque or to the Orthodox church. Yes, we fought against religion, but mostly Jehovah's Witnesses and Baptists. I was even at their meetings. It was difficult to get there, because they constantly changed their location. But we received information of who is going where, et cetera. Mind you, no one would be imprisoned for their beliefs. Imprisonment only happened when the law was broken. For example, we had a law that children under eighteen should not be drawn into the cult. . . . We actively campaigned [*agitirovali*], we told people that there is no God, that it is human morality that makes society, those kinds of things. And we asked them: "Why do you need this God? Don't you know how detrimental [*vrednyi*] all of that is?" That is how we worked, but the thing is that at that time there was order. Everyone had work. This [chaos] is what we got with your ideology, when money comes first. Nowadays people only think about making money, they don't care if what they sell is bad for people's health.

After the interview had ended we drank tea with cookies and talked about the changes in the city as well as her former colleagues. Many of them had started to teach about the history of religion instead of socialism. She looked dismissive, saying, "For me that doesn't work. Life is short, and I don't have time, I can't simply change my ideology." She then took a bottle of vodka from the cupboard and announced, "Let's conclude this meeting the Soviet way" (*po sovetskii*).

These briefly presented views significantly overlap. They agreed that atheism had disappeared to the extent that it had become rare to find self-proclaimed atheists, and that religious voices were being propagated instead of atheist ones. They connected these trends to the collapse of Soviet institutions and Soviet morality, but they disagreed as to whether this was a positive or negative development. Beyond these agreements and disagreements the three women emphasized different aspects or dimensions of "really existing" Soviet atheism.

The Issue of Substance

Does atheism have substance? In other words, should we read it as merely the absence of religion—that is, as *a*-theism—or as an ideological stance in its own right, athe-*ism*? The examples above suggest that both interpretations need to be considered.

The nonideology, or empty ideology, view came through most strongly in the comments of Olga, who had difficulty providing details when I prompted her to do so, suggesting that the topic never had any intrinsic value to her. This is not to say that she did not make an effort in her teaching. She filled the void of atheism by providing lively examples of the hypocrisy of religious leaders, and by emphasizing the progress of science. Along somewhat similar lines, Svetlana stressed that atheism was part of the larger project of socialism, and that as "the tenth thing," it derived value from that connection. The emphasis on science and the larger socialist project indicated that "atheism" did not have affective qualities in and of itself.

This "emptiness of atheism" creates a problem, because as long as it is centered on a void or absence it has trouble producing commitment. As atheist activist Madalyn Murray O'Hair said about atheism in North America, the problem is that "although [atheists are] numerous [they remain] unorganized and complacent" (cited in Martin 2007b, 220; Baggini 2009). Similarly, the humanists in Britain tend to present themselves as an unrecognized avant-garde for a silent majority of like-minded others (Engelke 2014; Matthew Engelke, pers. comm.). The situation was different in the state-socialist version of atheism. There, atheist organizations boasted huge membership, but especially toward the end of the Soviet period these were characterized by a weak internal structure behind a Potemkin-like facade (Peris 1998, 118–20). Officials and specialists were well aware of the indifference of both atheist activists and their audience. A telling example is provided by David Powell, citing a Soviet official who, in his speech at a conference of atheist specialists, exclaimed, in exasperation, "I repeat: it [religiosity] is a feeling, and you cannot fight it without instilling a counter feeling" (1967, 375).

The need to produce "counter feelings" may well be why atheisms the world over have a tendency to acquire "religious" characteristics. This is evident particularly in organized forms of atheism, where the original emphasis on reason and rationality or on "the absence of religion" is complemented by the celebration of heroes and exemplary men and women, by "sacred" symbols, and utopian visions of society. As Grace Davie (2012, 4) has suggested, "Communities of unbelief in each country form mirror images of [the existing religious] institutions." This "mirroring" works in two distinct ways, as can be seen in the Soviet case. On the one hand, there is the tendency to define atheism as the opposite of how specific versions of religions are being seen, and thus to stress the features of "rationality," "progress," and being "for the masses," all in contrast to the backwardness and oppressive nature of religion. On the other hand, though, there is a tendency for atheist organizations to manifest themselves, in Jesse Smith's words, as the "functional equivalent of organized religion" (2013, 92). Convenient Soviet examples are the Lenin and Stalin cults, the almost "religious" devotion that many Soviet citizens demonstrated to these leaders, and the emphasis on creating secular rituals that engaged with the big questions of life and death (see especially Lane 1981). Ironically, these "functional equivalents" suggest that atheism only becomes affective at the moment that it negates itself, when it is no longer an "a-theism" but a pseudo religion. This pseudoreligious fervor fizzled out in the late Soviet period, although Asel' still invoked it by saying, "We were also believers" back then—"Our God was Marxism, Leninism."[10] But although she spoke of Soviet atheism as a religion, in which communist prophets had taken over the place of Jesus and Muhammad, she also stressed that it was a vulgar and simplistic imitation of religion. Or as Tabyshalieva wrote, among the intelligentsia the cynical question emerged: "Did we have the pure atheism or did we perhaps [only] get its imitation?" (1993, 121).

Scientific atheism did not have an appeal in and of itself, but rather gained legitimacy, at least for some activists, by being part of a larger scheme. This came through most clearly in Svetlana's suggestion that antireligious struggle was "maybe the tenth thing," and her emphasis on the importance of the larger Soviet project. But when this larger scheme, the promised communist future, lost in credibility, there was very little to lean on. The resulting problem of indifference, of erosion from within, has been termed "a-atheism" by William van den Bercken, who suggested that this "fairly common phenomenon in Soviet society" was best described as "a form of secularization within the ideological monoculture, of removal of ideology from the personal sphere" (1985, 275).

The Issue of Difference

As mentioned earlier, atheism often reveals itself as an anti-theism. Soviet atheism gained momentum through the fight against organized religion. Atheist and antireligious fervor was at its height in the early decades of Soviet rule. Contested as these antireligious efforts were, the early members of the *bezbozhniki* (the communist league of the godless), the female Uzbek communists involved in the *hujum*, or unveiling campaigns (Kamp 2006), and the workers and peasants involved in the expropriation of religious buildings and properties across the USSR (Husband 2000) cannot be denied some measure of enthusiasm.[11] That is, atheism was a motivating force when it faced a clear adversary, and could present itself as part of a forward-moving project directed at a modern future.

The idea that atheist fervor is produced through opposition also emerged from the stories people told me about their own involvement in antireligious efforts in the late Soviet period. Recall Svetlana Iussupovna's insistence that she never went to fight against a mosque or Orthodox church but instead targeted the Jehovah's Witnesses and Baptists. She elaborated on the detrimental effects these "sects," as she called them, had on young children. A similar point was made, indirectly, by Asel' Kosobaeva, who found herself outraged when talking to Kyrgyz who were no longer Muslims but had become Baptists. The message speaking through this example was that certain forms of religiosity were too closely interwoven with the social and cultural fabric of late Soviet life to be seen as legitimate targets of antireligious interventions. Instead, the antireligious activists targeted unfitting elements such as Kyrgyz Baptists or the Jehovah's Witnesses. The point is that the antireligious position gained legitimacy and fervor at those moments when it was directed at a clearly identifiable adversary.

It was thus through identifying the problematic "Other" that antireligious rhetoric was likely to find wider resonance even in the late Soviet period. At some point I discussed with several middle-aged men their views of the local "unregistered Baptist" community living in Kokjangak. The Soviet media, schoolteachers, and other official communications had always portrayed these Baptists in an extremely negative light, using the derisive terms *sekta* (sect) and *fanatiki* (fanatics). Talking about this, Nurbek, one of my self-avowed not-religious acquaintances, remarked: "I never believed the stories that the Baptists would sacrifice one of their children on a special holiday and would then eat the child, I never believed that. But I did believe the stories that once a year they would retreat to partake in a secret sexual orgy." The anecdote was intentionally humorous, but also indicated that Nurbek used to perceive intense forms of self-avowed religiosity as being out of the ordinary—intriguing, abnormal—and, moreover, that he had internalized those aspects of antireligious propaganda that were in line with already-held fears, desires, and perhaps especially his (teenage) fantasies.

By contrast, when it came to the fight against versions of religion that were deemed legitimate, things were different. It is not accidental that Svetlana stressed that they never went to the (Orthodox) church or the mosque. The difficulties atheist activists experienced with regard to affiliation with Islam were also due to the fact that a boundary between religion and culture cannot be easily drawn. Although during the 1930s and 1950s, in particular, the Soviet regime had waged extensive antireligious campaigns in which imams were prosecuted and most mosques and madrassas were shut down, it had been far less successful in eradicating the many aspects of religious expression and identity that were part of everyday life. In fact, even while the Soviet regime successfully combated many public manifestations of religion, it ironically also encoded religious identities through its nationality politics. As Kemal Karpat has shown for Soviet Central Asia more generally, the appeal of newly created national categories derived (in part) from "the incorporation of many elements of the religious culture in the emerging 'national' cultures [which gave] the adherents of the latter a sense of the historical continuity, strength, and durability of their cultures" (1993, 416). Vice versa, the incorporation of religious elements in conceptualizations of ethnicity, nationality, and culture also enshrined the position of Islam. As a Soviet periodical noted, "The survivals of Islam often appear under the mask of national traditions" (Ro'i 1984, 34). Soviet authorities bemoaned this intertwining of religious and national affiliation, as in the following complaint of the *obkom* (province committee) secretary of Osh Province (*oblast*) in southern Kyrgyzstan: "Some people suggest that a person who observes Islamic rites demonstrates thereby 'respect' for his nation, and in deviating from them insults it" (cited ibid., 36).

By the end of the Soviet period, national identity was intimately tied to Muslimness, but a Muslimness that had been stripped of much of its "spiritual" content and was thereby made compatible with Soviet ideals (Shahrani 1995). Conversely, the processes allowed for an environment where self-avowed atheists could actively claim to be Muslims. This overlap between religion and culture has continued to inspire interesting points of view among the "not religious," such as the following statement of a middle-aged woman who used to be member of the Communist Party: "Look, we are atheists, but of course we all believe in God." She later elaborated: "We are atheists. Yes, we are Muslims, but let me explain. We are all Muslim people—Kazaks, Kyrgyz, Uzbeks, Turkmen, Tajiks. We were born Muslims. That's it" (quoted in McBrien and Pelkmans 2008, 87).

Disillusionment with the communist project is often—by and large correctly—attributed to the effect of a widening gap between the utopian communist vision and the reality of everyday Soviet life. But how does atheism fit into this picture? Soviet ideology was highly utopian, and the communist idea was accompanied by visions of healthy and affluent workers who achieved self-realization through their involvement in collective labor, and a new and modern age of technological achievements. Atheism, in itself, did not inspire such visions. Soviet leaders never *promised* atheism, and citizens did not desire atheism. The lack of a utopian dimension meant that it could not survive as a self-standing positive ideology. Its dependence on an Other meant that atheism (as anti-theism) worked only for as long as an external religious adversary could be identified, while attempts to instill "counter-feelings" from within resulted in pseudoreligious qualities that negated or compromised the atheist position. Sure, Soviet atheism continued to exist as part of the ideological state apparatus, embedded in a range of institutions, but disinterest and skepticism had corroded it from within long before the Soviet Union collapsed.

New Resonances of Soviet Atheism

As he had done on previous occasions, Kadyr expressed his perplexity of what he saw as people's gullibility, their propensity to buy into the "fairy tales" (*skazki*) of the imam and any of the new preachers. We were sitting, once again, on a grassy hill overlooking the town, this time accompanied by Bolot, one of Kadyr's oldest friends. Each of us holding a bottle of Baltika beer, we were sharing stories. "I am astonished that my neighbors believe this crap [*erunda*]," Kadyr repeated. Bolot agreed with him, but couldn't refrain from mentioning that in the early 1990s he and Kadyr had once traveled all the way to the city of Kokand (located two hundred kilometers to the southwest) to see a spiritual healer. We laughed, as one does with beer in hand, about the various events in Kokand, including Bolot's momentary belief that drinking some kind of magical potion was going to heal his chronic headaches. . . . After a short silence, half a cigarette long, Kadyr said, now in a pensive mood, "I know, but those were different times . . . everyone was confused back then." Their visit to a famous spiritual healer was remembered as having been about curiosity, experimentation, and momentary confusion, after which they had come to their senses. By contrast, people who had started to devote themselves to strict interpretations of Islam or Christianity were in Kadyr's view of a different sort; they had become "fanatics."

Earlier I mentioned that Kadyr had never cared for scientific atheism, and had been happy to ridicule the predictable rhetoric of antireligious activists. At the same time, though, his views expressed ambivalence. With the Soviet system no longer in existence, with religious leaders expressing their opinion without being challenged, and with religious symbolism becoming more conspicuous in the public sphere, the disappearance of atheism was no longer a straightforwardly positive change. In other words, it seemed that the contextual changes led Kadyr and Bolot to reconsider their position. As Bolot put it: "Much of what the communists taught us was right, but at the time we didn't appreciate it." This idea resonates with the key analytical problem of this chapter: the problem of an empty ideology, which produced indifference as long as it was the dominant, official narrative, yet started to be appreciated after its structures collapsed. The contrarian quality of atheism—deriving energy from its antagonistic counterpart religion—regained relevance after the collapse of the Soviet Union, with the ironic result that the "not religious" appeared to be defending something that they had not desired when it existed. The question that therefore needs to be answered is: How did the oppositional and relational dimensions of atheism become reconfigured after 1991?

One of the challenges faced by the "not religious" was that their conduct was no longer always sufficient to qualify as Muslim. During Soviet times it had been a sine qua non that Kyrgyz men would drink vodka (see also Khalid 2006, 1); alcohol consumption was an important ingredient in assertions of masculinity and was closely entwined with ideas of hospitality. Although most men continued these practices, they were increasingly criticized for doing so. Women faced other challenges. When once visiting school number 4 with my Kyrgyz colleague Himia, we briefly talked to some teenagers who were loitering in the school yard. One of these young men confronted Himia, telling her that she should not wear trousers and should wear a head scarf. It was an exceptional and very confronting occasion to Himia, not only because her Muslimness was being questioned, but also because age hierarchies were publicly being violated.

There were other challenges to established patterns of engagement with Islam as well. If during the Soviet period it was generally assumed that only the very old would pray (and rarely in a mosque), by the mid-2000s not only larger numbers of old men but especially many young men and boys would come to the Friday prayers and the study sessions organized by Imam Talant. He also tried to convince middle-aged men to pray, but they turned out to be insensitive to his arguments. As the imam complained in a conversation with me: "The problem is that they still have an atheist mind-set. They always have excuses, and they always think that they know it better, telling me that the Kyrgyz had never prayed in mosques. But this is not about being Kyrgyz, this is about Islam. Islam is one and Kyrgyz is another."

Imam Talant was not the only one who attempted to disentangle religion and culture, and thus to undo a connection that had been reinforced under Soviet rule. Local Tablighi circles became increasingly active in the 2000s. They not only invited inhabitants to start praying, but also addressed false conceptions of Islam in their teachings, and criticized, for example, funerals and weddings, which were deemed un-Islamic. These issues were reported across the region. McBrien, for example, documents how newly pious Muslims started to transform life-cycle rituals into "religiously pure" events in the nearby town of Bazar-Korgon. By abolishing "traditional" wedding parties, prohibiting serving alcohol, reinforcing gender segregation, and inviting wedding speakers, these newly pious Muslims challenged the formerly agreed-on notions of what was Islamic and what was not (McBrien 2006). Such innovations worked to disconnect being Muslim from being Kyrgyz, stressing the supranational character of Islam rather than its relation to culture and national identity. But although such newly pious assertions made significant headway in several settlements, in Kokjangak it was still a relatively marginal phenomenon. Residents explained this by referring to the town's history as a mining town—a former beacon of socialist modernity—and that therefore the mind-set of its inhabitants was more "cultured" and modern. For example, they pointed out that whereas they had been to "Islamic" funerals in other settlements, in Kokjangak such funerals had taken place only a couple of times, and these had been talked badly about.

One important legacy of "atheism" is that it provided citizens with a vocabulary to respond to religious authorities. My acquaintances drew on a repertoire of received wisdom, much of which had its roots in Soviet times. Kadyr, for example, several times quoted the Kyrgyz saying that "one should listen to what the mullah says, but not do as he does" as a way to underline that a lot of this self-avowed religiosity was simple pretense. At other times he pointed at one of the first post-Soviet imams, who had received money to build a mosque through a foreign charity, but instead used it to furnish his own house. This atheist vocabulary was also evident in the usage of terms such as "sects" and "fanatics" to refer to unhealthy forms of religiosity. In this way, they were trying to restore the boundary between the religious and the secular, which in their view had been trespassed by unwelcome assertions of religiosity in the public sphere.

Kadyr's weariness about new religiosity was also informed by developments across the border in Uzbekistan. On more than one occasion he told me that in his opinion Uzbekistan's president, Islom Karimov, was doing the right thing in repressing religion. "If Karimov would not repress the fanatics, then those Uzbeks would reinstate sharia in no time, and we would have an Islamic state as a neighbor within no time." Kadyr felt the situation was a bit better in Kyrgyzstan: "Of course, our people are less fanatic than Uzbeks ... but still." Such fears may have been informed by negative ethnic stereotyping, but the fear was real enough. Kadyr was convinced that religion should be controlled, and he opposed the idea of freedom of religion. "Maybe such freedom is a good thing in Western Europe, but here it is dangerous. Our people are not suited for it." He continued by criticizing the presence of the small group of Tablighis in town, asserting that "they don't work and they can only think about religion—they always tell you the same thing."

Kadyr's negative feelings about excessive religiosity intensified particularly when his two sons (twins who were twelve years old in 2008) started to display interest in Islam, and secretly joined some of the other boys from the neighborhood in meetings organized at the mosque by the imam and several Tablighis. When Kadyr found out about this, he gave his sons a stern lecture and forbade them to go again; but sensing this might not be sufficient (at least for the twin who was most intrigued), he made sure to keep his sons busy with domestic tasks when the Tablighi meetings were taking place.

Inhabitants like Kadyr who saw themselves as "not religious" were clearly disturbed by new assertions of devotion. In conversation they would often express opinions similar to those of Kadyr, and stereotype the Tablighis—as well as other new religious groups such as Pentecostals—as zombies, fanatics, and extremists. It was also clear that the encounters with the imam and with Tablighis were discomforting precisely because "the truth" had become instable. With antireligious discourse having lost the institutional backing it had enjoyed during Soviet times, attempts to discredit the authoritative basis of newly active religious movements had become even more important. For example, "not religious" inhabitants insisted that leaders of new religious movements used brainwashing techniques and offered payments to attract followers. McBrien offers some valuable observations from the aforementioned town of Bazar-Korgon. Toward the end of Ramadan 2003, members of the Islamist group Hizb ut-Tahrir put up fliers around town that invited Muslims to follow the "true path." McBrien discussed the episode with a fifty-year-old schoolteacher, who denounced the messages and aims of the group. "He called the group 'bad' and 'dangerous,' and labeled its members 'extremists.' At the end of his diatribe [he] furiously remarked that those who had physically tacked the signs up around town must have been paid to do so. Why else would they have been involved in such activities, he mused aloud" (McBrien and Pelkmans 2008, 92). What is clear from these examples is that people who depicted themselves as "not religious" became infused with "atheist" energy when confronted with a new adversary.

Further Reflections

Atheism, to the extent it had existed during Soviet times, lost the institutional backing it once enjoyed. Even the term itself tended to be avoided by those who defined themselves as "not religious." But this does not mean that atheist ideas completely evaporated. Remnants of atheism continued to exist, and lent force to a contrarian position, either to discredit religious groups or to doubt and ridicule religious claims. As I will discuss in subsequent chapters, many of the faith-driven movements continued to wage discursive battles, not so much against atheism as an ideology, but against the notions that emerged in its wake.

In this chapter I focused on inhabitants who referred to themselves as being "not close to religion" or as "not religious" Muslims. On the one hand they denounced Soviet atheism, but this was accompanied by a fear of what was seen as excessive religiosity, something they identified in many of the "new" religious currents gaining ground in the country starting in the late 1990s. Their criticisms of "excessive religiosity" inadvertently linked back to Soviet atheist ideology, as was already evident in Svetlana's, at least partly affirmative, allusion to "the opium of the people."

In a previous cowritten publication (McBrien and Pelkmans 2008, 98–99) I used an example that I still find telling. In 2002 Kyrgyzstan's daily newspaper *Vechernii Bishkek* published a series of articles on the presumed detrimental effects of both Christian and Islamic "extremism." One of these articles (March 19, 2002) incorrectly cited Marx: "Karl Marx was right after all when he announced: 'Religion is the opium of the people! Sweet, intoxicating, and mysterious. In small quantities it is medicine. In large quantities it is poison.'" Clearly the newspaper's editors viewed the success of new religious movements as an undesirable and dangerous development, one that poisoned the youth and turned them into spiritual drug addicts. Marx of course never made a distinction between the curative small dose and the addictive large dose of religion. Instead he criticized the soothing quality of much institutionalized religion, while acknowledging the transformative potential of religious movements such as, for example, Lutheranism.[12] Oblivious to such nuances, the newspaper twisted Marx's views through their drug metaphor in order to defend what was called "folk" or "liberal" Islam, while depicting the new religious movements as dangerous and detrimental. The views presented in this chapter revealed a similar logic. Clearly, the "not religious" were afraid of the transformative potential of religion, and their responses were stark instances of the need to distance oneself from the new religiosity. Marx had returned with a twist.

In a further play on the drug metaphor one could even postulate that the "not religious" feared that these religions were in fact not a "downer" that relaxes and pacifies as opium does, but rather an "upper" that energizes and emboldens; in essence, they worried that "religion is the cocaine of the people." By contrast, Soviet "atheism" always had difficulties in becoming an upper, and lacked the energizing potential of cocaine. It was only in response to an adversary that atheist thought gained momentum. This need for an adversary is, as we will see in later chapters, also present in other ideologies. But because it lacked a utopian dimension, the tendency was particularly pronounced in the case of scientific atheism.

To recall, Althusser argued that ideology obtains part of its strength from a double-mirror connection in which subjects are pulled in by the "voice of ideology" in a process of mutual recognition. But because this "voice" was compromised in the case of Soviet atheism, it started to disintegrate and erode while it was hegemonic, yet gained momentum when the mirror was directed not toward the (here nonexistent) unique Subject, but toward the external "Object," a process not of identification but of differentiation. Using Yurchak's terms, when the "hegemony of form" collapsed, elements of atheist content, parts of its constative meaning, reappeared. Or, as an earlier presented voice from Kokjangak suggested in less abstract terms: "Much of what the communists told us was right, but at the time we did not appreciate it."

This suggests that the legacy of the atheist project and the continued existence of unbelief should not be brushed under the rug. The remnants of atheism continued to be found in the ways in which those who are "not religious" approached the world. But they did so hesitantly, as they were struggling to find a position between the extremes of Soviet atheism and new religiosity. For those who were "not religious," uncertainty remained about what is true, about what is fact and what is fantasy.

4

Walking the Truth in Islam with the Tablighi Jamaat

In April 2009 I took part in a three-day *dawat*, or proselytizing tour, of the Tablighi Jamaat, a conservative Islamic piety movement, which has made significant inroads into Kyrgyzstan since the 1990s.[1] One afternoon our fellowship (*jamaat*) was seated around a low table in the courtyard behind the mosque, eating a warm lunch. We were talking about spiritual affairs when Maksat, who was on his third *dawat* asked, "Is it true what they say, that when you go to heaven there will be twelve hundred virgins waiting?" Nur-Islam, a middle-aged Dungan[2] and the *amir*, or leader, of our fellowship, responded, "There will be many virgins, and what is more, every one of those virgins will be more beautiful than the most beautiful woman you have ever seen in your life. And your own wife, she will be the most gorgeous one of all." Around the table tongues were clicking. Some of the men expressed looks of affirmation, others of anticipation. Not wishing to confront what to me came across as sexism, yet unable to listen quietly, I interjected, "How is that even possible? I mean, which man would be able to satisfy so many women?" It turned out to be a naive question. Nur-Islam responded in a serious demeanor, "Well, you should understand that in heaven your manly powers will be multiplied as well."

Sex and women were recurrent topics of conversation among *dawatchis* (participants in *dawat*, or "travelers"), and this particular episode continues to stand out when I think of the three *dawats* in which I participated. One reason for its memorable nature is that the topic made me uncomfortable, as I was unable to join in the fascination. Another reason was the seriousness and detail with which the virgin story was discussed among the men. Indeed, what fascinated me most was that these ideas momentarily attained a level of reality I had not expected. I was surprised, not only because of my own biases, but also because most of my acquaintances in Kyrgyzstan had only ever spoken of "the virgins" as a kind of joke, if at all.[3] The fantasy did, however, connect with locally widespread ideas and practices. While for young unmarried women the ideal of chastity is valued highly, it is commonly accepted and expected that married men have as many "girlfriends" as their financial and social position allows. The "reality of the virgins" did not emerge out of thin air but was richly connected to ideas of masculinity, sexuality, and worldly success.

In this chapter I focus on Tablighi techniques to make and keep ideas relevant, believable, and embodied. Although we tend to think of ideologies as configurations of ideas, the ideas that make up ideologies do not necessarily travel as a package; they often move in fragments and bits. New ideologies are rarely accepted at once; their internalization can be a haphazard process, characterized by intensification, deflation, and (partial) evaporation. That is, their trajectories are endowed with a pulsating quality. This tends to be particularly visible when ideologies are "new," that is, when they are encountered "as new" in adulthood instead of being acquired through upbringing and socialization from an early age onward.

The external observer does not usually notice this pulsating quality; and especially when access is limited to one moment in time, this may result in depictions of belief and unbelief as fixed states.[4] By contrast, movements such as the Tablighi Jamaat are cognizant of the pulsating quality of faith and have devised their own strategies to combat the dissipation of conviction.[5] Their central energizing practice is *dawat*, which can be provisionally translated as "proselytizing tour." Ideally Tablighis go on *dawat* for one evening a week, three consecutive days each month, a forty-day *dawat* each year, and a four-month *dawat* once in a lifetime. On three-day *dawats* (the most common form in Kyrgyzstan), participants travel to a mosque other than their own in groups of six to ten men. During these *dawats* the three aspects of traveling, male bonding, and storytelling produce an effect of intensification, which allows access to levels of experience that tend to remain untouched in everyday life. Hence, though the Urdu term *dawat* stems from the Arabic term *da'wa*, which means "invitation," and in the Tablighi context can be translated as "proselytizing tour," the spiritual effect is foremost on the *dawatchis* themselves instead of the villagers and townspeople they encounter and invite to follow the same path. For the travelers, *dawat* offers an opportunity to learn, to translate loosely held ideas into an Islamic vocabulary, and to consolidate these in practice and routine. The embodied truth that is thus produced does not, however, necessarily last long after the *dawatchis* return home.

Dawatchis in Kyrgyzstan

The historical trajectory of the Tablighi Jamaat has often been described, starting from its origins in northern India in the 1920s, to its increasingly transnational profile from the 1950s onward, culminating in the late twentieth century in its recognition as one of the largest Islamic piety or renewal movements in the world(Metcalf 1993, 2002; Masud 2000a; Gaborieau 2000). Close-up analyses of the Tablighi Jamaat tend to be frustrated by the movement's public silence.[6] The movement avoids making public statements and discourages its adherents from talking to journalists. In Kyrgyzstan this low profile meant that many participants were unaware of the name Tablighi Jamaat when they first became involved. The term more commonly used by both insiders and outsiders was *dawatchi*, which refers to people who go on *dawat*. Unawareness of the "official" name was even true for Kanat, who had become involved in Tablighi activities when studying abroad. He became a *dawatchi* after returning to Kyrgyzstan but only discovered that "*dawat* is the same thing as Tablighi Jamaat" when he asked an *alim* (scholar of Islam) about the connection. Ignorance of the name has nothing to do with secrecy but everything to do with organizational features. Because of the Tablighi's decentralized structure and the emphasis on engagement rather than affiliation—there are no registered members—the "official" name is not all that relevant.

Dawat first appeared in Kyrgyzstan in 1992, when Tablighis from Pakistan traveled to the country. According to the story, when they arrived at the central mosque in Bishkek, no one including the mufti understood their motives or background except for one Kyrgyz Muslim who had spent time in Pakistan. This man ended up taking the visiting Tablighis to his hometown of Balykchi, which subsequently became known as the birthplace of *dawat* in Kyrgyzstan (Toktogulova 2014, 7). In the early years the movement remained small and was barely noticed, but this started to change around the turn of the millennium. The first time I met a small group of *dawatchis* was in 2003 in a mosque in Karakol (northeastern Kyrgyzstan) while doing research on conversion to Christianity. I asked them their opinion of evangelical missionaries and of Muslims converting to Christianity. Their answer was straightforward: those Kyrgyz had never been real Muslims; Christians had simply done more mission work than Muslims in the 1990s; this was changing now that Muslims such as themselves were becoming more active in calling people closer to Islam. As suggested by this answer, the rise of Tablighi activity in Kyrgyzstan was in part a response to Christian evangelization, just like in the 1920s the movement sprang from its founder's desire to counteract Christian and Hindi proselytizing in northwest India (Masud 2000a, xxvi; 2000b, 7).

Because of the absence of formal membership it is not possible to provide precise numbers, but by 2007 an estimated ten thousand people were involved in Tablighi activities.[7] Several *dawatchis* claimed that in 2005, often mentioned as the movement's heyday in Kyrgyzstan to date, some two hundred *jamaats* ("fellowships" of six to ten men) left Bishkek each Friday to start their three-day *dawat*. A former *dawatchi* said: "There was like a *jamaat* in every minibus leaving the capital." Though these are probably overestimates, *dawatchis* certainly became a familiar sight throughout the country. Explaining this relative success is not my primary aim here. However, a discussion of the movement's advance in the region will lay the groundwork for exploration of my central theme: how commitment and conviction are temporarily produced.

The Tablighi advance in Central Asia has been uneven, making significant inroads into Kyrgyzstan and Kazakhstan but failing to do so in Turkmenistan, Tajikistan, and Uzbekistan (see Balci 2012). This may be unsurprising given that the Tablighi Jamaat is banned as an extremist group in Uzbekistan, Tajikistan, and Turkmenistan (and more recently

Kazakhstan). However, the pattern is replicated within Kyrgyzstan in the sense that Uzbeks (who make up a sizable 12% of the population) hardly take part in Tablighi activities.[8] This is counterintuitive because Uzbeks are locally depicted as more religious than Kyrgyz in that they more strictly observe the pillars of Islam.[9] Success among the "less religious" is also geographically visible in Kyrgyzstan where the Tablighis have attracted more participants in the locally depicted "secular" north than the "Islamic" south of the country. A Tablighi *alim* (scholar) reflected on these patterns when I interviewed him:

> Dawat used to be active in Uzbekistan and Tajikistan in the 1990s, but [the Tablighis there] made a mistake. They became involved in politics, while our position needs to be absolutely apolitical. So then Allah took [*dawat*] away from these countries. There is another thing. Uzbeks have traditionally paid more attention to religious education, to going to the mosque, et cetera. And once you have gone down one path it is very difficult to return and start anew. The Kyrgyz were different. They were like a blank slate.

The point about the reverse correlation between doctrinal knowledge and the appeal of Tablighi methods resonated in the following condescending view of an Uzbek man living in Kyrgyzstan: "Why would I listen to those *dawatchis* who only know the basics of Islam?!"[10] In short, the Tablighi's uneven progress in Central Asia and the locally offered interpretations suggest that the relative success in Kyrgyzstan is due not only to a favorable political environment but also to the focus on learning through participation, which makes it particularly attractive to people who are interested yet unschooled in Islamic doctrine.[11]

Another geographic pattern is that the Tablighi Jamaat has a larger following in urban than in rural areas. A likely reason is that *dawat* offers a form of male bonding that fills a real need in post-Soviet urban contexts, and several *dawatchis* told me that through *dawat* they reconnected with former school friends. The kind of "outdoor" traveling of *dawat* is also more likely to attract urban than rural young men. Almost all urban travelers (those aged thirty-plus) commented that *dawat* reminded them of the Soviet pioneer and Komsomol camps, when they would leave the city to spend time in nature, with only the most basic facilities available.

If the Soviet legacy provides clues for why the Tablighis find resonance among Kyrgyz urban men, this legacy also clarifies why they fail to pro- duce the same response among urban women. In fact, there are hardly any all-women *jamaats* that travel (accompanied by a related male) beyond their own settlement. Occasionally special *dawats* are organized for mar- ried couples (called *masturat dawat*), but these are few and far between. First, as an organization the Tablighi Jamaat is less accessible to women, and most involved women are so through their husbands. Second, Tablighi ideas of proper gender behavior do not translate easily to the post-Soviet Kyrgyz context. The (university-educated) spouse of a *dawatchi* expressed her view of the Tablighi Jamaat to me in a dismissive and condescend- ing tone of voice: "*Never* will I join them. Their idea of a woman is to be submissive, to serve her husband, and to stay at home with the children." Such ideas clash, not only with seventy years of Soviet discourse on female emancipation, but also with the fact that most Kyrgyz urban women have jobs outside the domestic sphere. To self-declared modern women, the increasingly public presence of conservative Islamic movements is worri- some (Heyat 2004).[12] The perspective of my male Tablighi acquaintances on this issue was captured best in a joke that circulated among them: "The largest obstacle to *dawat* in Kyrgyzstan is Kyrgyz women."

It is not only among educated women that negative opinions about Tablighis can be found. The same was true for many men and women who describe themselves as "not religious." One of my acquaintances in Kokjangak told me: "They dress like fanatics [*fanatiki*], and, really, it is impossible to have a normal conversation with them. They only talk about religion, religion, religion [Kyrgyz, *deen, deen, deen*]." The director of the Kyrgyz Committee of Religious Affairs added his own personal view to his ready-made stump speech about respecting religious freedom when I interviewed him in the summer of 2011:

You know, Kyrgyz people are horse riders. When a boy is born, the first thing he learns is to ride a horse. And horse riders need to wear trousers. This is deeply ingrained in our culture. We were the ones who introduced trousers to Europe! [disapprovingly] Now these Tablighis import dressing codes from Pakistan, walking around in long robes! This is completely alien to our people.

The emphasis on garments illustrates that the Tablighi advance is threatening to notions of Kyrgyz culture precisely by reconfiguring "cultural" elements into "religious" ones, as was also discussed in chapter 3.[13]

Although some of the practices are indeed of foreign origin, the Tablighis are not a foreign-driven presence. In fact, the decentered nature of the movement means that notwithstanding its foreign roots, it is a local movement and one that, by the late 2000s, had established many connections with secular and religious authorities in Kyrgyzstan. Of these connections, those with the muftiate were especially valuable, because they lent security and legitimacy to Tablighi activities. The muftiate of Kyrgyzstan has a Dawat and Propagation Department that deals with different forms of *da'wa*, including Tablighi activities. The department issues permissions to *dawatchis* to go on a forty-day tour (after submitting several documents, including a written agreement from their spouse), which need to be shown to the imams of receiving mosques and to the police when requested to do so. The involvement of the muftiate does not mean, however, that all its clergy are favorably disposed to the Tablighi Jamaat. One of the four deputy muftis expressed to me the following critical view, meanwhile attempting to reappropriate the term *dawat* by stressing its original meaning of "invitation":

> These Tablighis should remember that the foremost *dawatchi* is the mufti himself; I and my colleagues, we are the second-foremost *dawatchis*. To carry out *dawat* does not require traveling around. What kind of *dawat* is it anyway when you leave your family hungry? We are not against the Tablighis, but there is no need to be overly protective of them. And some of their ways, such as their clothing, are harmful to the faith because it scares people away.[14]

Once again we encounter ambivalent attitudes toward the Tablighis. Their non-Kyrgyz appearance is thoroughly disliked, while as Muslims they are treated with respect; they encounter distrust among secular (and religious) authorities,[15] but also have multiple connections within the establishment. Such ambivalence also characterizes the relationship between the Tablighis and the law. A 2009 law against proselytism implied that the Tablighi practice of *gasht*—in which *dawatchis* go from door to door to invite people to the mosque—would henceforth be illegal. However, the *dawatchis* with whom I discussed the issue were untroubled by this law, or as one of them put it: "This law is intended [to restrict proselytization by] Jehovah's Witnesses. But it is different for us, because this is a Muslim country." Again, this does not mean that people generally welcome the Tablighis, but rather that their activities are condoned. When asked, the deputy director of the State Committee of Religious Affairs admitted that the law is not enforced in the case of the Tablighis, and justified this by saying that the population largely rejects them anyway: "When they knock on someone's door, the usual response is 'Be gone!' [Russian, *poshel ty*]."

The Tablighis are, to borrow a famous phrase from Turner, "neither here nor there, they are betwixt and between the positions arrayed by law, custom, convention, and ceremonial" (1969, 95). They are Muslim but of a different kind. They look foreign, but most Tablighis are Kyrgyz. Their message is both attractive and repulsive: the emphasis on learning through doing and the sense of fraternity have appeal to a significant group; their mode of conduct and theology are reprehensible to many others. This liminal position generates an aura of exclusivity and sense of purpose, lending their mission importance and uniqueness. It also contributes to the intensity of spiritual experience, as Turner intimated when he wrote about the blend of "lowliness and sacredness, of homogeneity and comradeship" that often arises in conditions of liminality (1969, 96). These characteristics are applicable to the movement as a whole, but the temporal dimension, the "moment in and out of time" (Turner 1969), reveals itself particularly clearly in the practice of *dawat*.

The Route There

After the Friday prayers in August 2009, approximately twenty-five men gathered at the mosque in a Bishkek neighborhood.[16] It was one of four mosques in Bishkek serving as sending points for *dawat*. Several men were wearing the white robe that makes Tablighis instantly recognizable, though the majority were dressed in everyday clothes. Most of the men sported beards, or had started growing them, an indicator of prolonged involvement. Over the next few hours, more men arrived, until at 4:00 p.m. the *jamaats* (fellowships) needed to be formed. This was first done informally, after which two coordinators ensured that all fellowships had a proper composition. They moved several men around so as to obtain a good spread of age and experience in each *jamaat*, and to ensure that the travelers would be able to communicate effectively with each other, either in Kyrgyz or Russian.

After this process was completed each *jamaat* needed to select its *amir*, or leader. This can be a delicate issue because potential leaders need to present their experience while retaining a modest deportment. After all, Tablighi etiquette says that "one must not expect nor insist on the acceptance of his suggestion" (Masud 2000b, 28). The procedure began with a round of introductions in which each traveler mentioned previous *dawat* participation. The more experienced travelers used the opportunity to comment on the values of *dawat* and thereby allow others to assess their suitability for leadership. Subsequently each traveler was asked to point to the person they deemed most suitable for the position of *amir*. In our group a young Kyrgyz man received the largest number of votes, only slightly beating a more senior Kyrgyz man. This slightly awkward situation was solved by splitting our *jamaat* of twelve into a Kyrgyz- and a Russian-language *jamaat*, and adding a few others from a third group. The Russian-language *jamaat*, of which I became part, was a heterogeneous mix of three Kyrgyz, two Tatars, one Uyghur, and me. The Kyrgyz-language groups were more ethnically homogeneous, with only one (Kyrgyz-speaking) Russian joining their ranks.

After the members of our *jamaat* had agreed to contribute 100 KGS (two dollars) each, our *amir* made a phone call to the *rukh jamaat* (head office), situated elsewhere in Bishkek, which coordinates the travel destinations. The groups' destinations are decided on the basis of the collected sum of money, the availability of a vehicle, and the even distribution of Tablighi visits to all villages and urban neighborhoods. Our fellowship had a car at its disposal, and we found ourselves being sent to a village located thirty kilometers west of Bishkek. When getting ready to depart everyone turned off their mobile phones—*dawatchis* are expected to sever all contact with friends and relatives for the duration of *dawat*. From here on, the *dawatchis* submit themselves to the leadership of the *amir* (see also Tozy 2000, 168).[17]

Despite my initial skepticism, it turned out that a three-door Toyota seats seven grown men. Packed together, with one of us repeating *zikr* (remembrance of God), others exchanging stories and anecdotes from previous *dawats*, and me listening to it all with my cheek pressed against the window, we reached our destination one hour later. The mosque was a transformed Soviet House of Culture (*Dom Kul'tury*), an inversion of the early Soviet practice to turn mosques into barns, sheds, and houses of culture. Both then and now the buildings continue to exude the atmosphere of their previous incarnations. If mosques-turned-sheds preserved an aura that invited respect and care, this House of Culture-turned-mosque had not entirely cast off its Soviet past either. Its dilapidated condition indicated villagers' indifference. Not long after our arrival the local imam appeared. He agreed to us staying in the mosque and promised to lead the two evening prayers.

The "route there" set in motion a process of detachment and separation from everyday life that allows for the formation of what Victor Turner calls *communitas*: a "generalized social bond . . . of equal individuals who submit together to the general authority of ritual elders" (1969, 96). These liminal aspects are core features of *dawat*. To quote Muhammad Khalid Masud, *dawat* is travel in the sense of both migration and withdrawal in which "one temporarily migrates from *dunya* (worldly pursuits) to *din* (religious concerns)" (2000a, xvi). The temporal and social conventions that govern everyday life are suspended during this period.

During the three days of *dawat* the men are not supposed to leave the mosque and its courtyard, except when authorized to do so by the *amir*. The rhythm and pace of life are altered, with only the prayer times remaining the same. There are time slots for going on *gasht* to invite people to the mosque, for studying, for receiving instructions about proper conduct, and for preparing food. Most of these activities are loosely structured, and leave much time for individual prayer, conversation, and resting. The men clearly valued being able to rest from their demanding ordinary lives. They took naps during the day and carried out their assigned tasks at a relaxed pace. Several compared being on *dawat* to being on holidays.

The plan for the day is decided at a meeting, or council (*mashvara*), each morning, during which the *amir* assigns tasks and roles to the *dawatchis*.[18] Assignments take into consideration level of experience and religious knowledge. For example, the *baian*, or sermon, after the midday prayers[19] is given by the more experienced *dawatchis*, while novices are asked to repeat the *zikr* (remembrance of God) for the benefit of the entire *dawat*. All travelers, except those who are very old, take turns being *kyzmat* (helper), charged with preparing food during one of the three days, tasks that in everyday life are considered female ones. Another traveler acts as the treasurer, taking responsibility for the necessary purchases related to transportation and food. During study sessions the more experienced *dawatchis* teach novices the pronunciation of *suras* and explain the six basic tenets of the Tabligh.[20]

These leveling techniques produce a sense of inclusion, equality, and companionship. The *dawatchis* cooperate in the basic activities of food preparation, engage as teachers and students, and learn intimate details about each other while sleeping together in one room and washing themselves side by side. Maksat stressed these aspects while we were smoking cigarettes just outside the mosque territory: "For me this is like the *lager* [camp]. When you arrive at the mosque you never know what to expect, you need to make do with the few available things. We buy some basic food and that is it. And yet nowhere does food taste as good as on *dawat*."[21]

To stick with Turner's vocabulary, the described egalitarian and pre-structural bonds facilitated the production of commitment and the embodiment of knowledge. But what gave it coherence and direction was the liminal experience. The temporal and spatial dimensions of *dawat* fenced it off from ordinary life, while the tensions with the outside world contributed to a sense of exclusivity and purpose. Beyond that, *dawat*, in its literal meaning of invitation, is all about straddling this boundary between inside and outside, which is revealed with particular clarity in the practice of *gasht*. *Gasht* refers to making rounds through the village in a small group consisting of a leader (*amir*), a speaker (*mutakalim*), and a guide from the locality (*zahbar*), going from door to door to invite men to come to the mosque. This practice of walking is aimed outwardly at drawing other people to Islam, but it is also an exercise in being a good Muslim.

Although Rashid Sultanovich had never been on *dawat* before, during his first *gasht* he was made speaker (*mutakalim*). At first he stumbled over his words, but using suggestions from the others he had his message more or less ready when approaching the fifth house:

> Good afternoon. I am Rashid Sultanovich, and with me are my brothers from Bishkek. As you know, it is very important to pray regularly and to follow the Prophet's way. Therefore we have come to invite you to the mosque to listen to the *baian* [sermon]).

Such encounters are often unsuccessful in the conventional sense. Only in a few of the encounters that I observed was the invitation accepted and followed up by the invitee actually showing up at the mosque. The far more common response was for the addressee to wait until the speaker has finished, and then either briskly express disinterest or politely decline the invitation. Such negative and evasive responses were not seen as problematic by the *dawatchis*; according to the Tablighi code, "the duty of the preacher ends with the communication of the message" (Masud 2000a, xxi).

Moreover, unsuccessful attempts had their own significance for the *dawatchis*, as the following example shows. After leaving the mosque with our four-person *gasht*, we were walking through the lush village street. Rashid and the guide were in front, with me and *amir* Seyit following in a second row. Seyit was marveling at the trees, and explained how each tree, each twig, and even each of the thousands of leaves had been individually shaped by God. He explained, "Everything around us has its purpose, its meaning, all willed by Allah." He continued by telling me and the others: "When you are on *gasht*, you are making traces through the village, which are like the footsteps of angels. . . . What we are doing is spinning a web of trails that have positive energy and can be picked up by those who come after us." In this spiritually charged environment the footsteps and trails woven by the *dawatchis* were seen as having the potential to transform the place. In a world that is saturated with the visible and invisible signs of the sacred and that is brimming with divine purpose, failure as such does not exist.

I have suggested that the intensification effect partly derives from "internal sharing," for which the ingredients are offered by *dawat*. This intensity also relies on a sense of exclusivity, produced through an "external facing," as illustrated by the negative and ambivalent encounters during the *gasht*, or village walks. The walks also show the importance of making the experiences meaningful, and storytelling plays an essential role in this. Indeed, what pervades all *dawat* activities are stories: anecdotes from previous *dawats*, religious messages, and interpretations of what is happening: the stories energize the *dawatchis*, invigorate their experience, and animate the landscape.

Enchanting Stories

A Tablighi acquaintance who accompanied me on several interviews told me with a laugh: "As you see, it is not easy to interview *dawatchis*; they talk too much."[22] Most of my questions remained indeed unanswered, but listening to their stories was all the more revealing. So after I had joined this acquaintance on several *dawats*, he told others: "His approach to research is a bit unconventional. He rarely asks questions, he just listens to what people have to say."

Stories are essential for meaningful living. In his book about Serbia in the early 1990s, Mattijs van de Port writes that he was struck by "everyone's complete reliance on a story, a story that can give meaning, direction and purpose to (certain aspects of) life" (1998, 29). He refers to this as "narrated/narrating reality" (*verhaalde werkelijkheid*) a term that suggests the inseparability between the world and experience (1994, 50–56; 1998, 50–52). In other words, stories do more than reflect and refract the world; they also shape lived reality, and do so by engaging the listener as well as the speaker. Rane Willerslev suggests that stories can be "a 'magical' tool for 'humanizing' hunters" (2007, 165), and according to Susan Harding (1987) it is through talking and telling stories that evangelical Baptists convert others. Stories are an important part of what constitutes experience, and they are tools for convincing others and self of what is true, important, or right.

In the case of the Tablighis stories were important venues by which *dawat* success was produced. Marc Gaboriau writes that Tablighi literature "is always anxious to proclaim that the preaching tours obtained wonderful results" (2000, 136). Or as *amir* Nur Islam put it to our fellowship, during *dawat* one should talk only about religion (*deen*) and focus on the positive, rather than allow Satan-inspired (*shaitan*) negativity. Metcalf stresses the centrality of stories for the Tablighi movement, which "engage the listener, . . . not only intellectually but emotionally" (1993, 593) and aim to achieve "experiential, not intellectual understanding" (1996, 110).

This section tries to understand how, through stories, such emotional connections and experiential understandings are produced. According to Geertz (1973, 100) "There are at least three points where chaos—a tumult of events which lack not just interpretations but interpretability—threatens to break in upon man." His three points, or limits, are those pertaining to the mind, the body, and the soul, or in his words: "at the limits of his analytic capacities, at the limits of his powers of endurance, and at the limits of his moral insight." These limits, which are obviously intertwined, also surfaced in stories told by Tablighis. The "limits of analytic capacity" resonated in stories that conveyed awe about the Creation and the occurrence of miracles. The "limits of power and endurance," referring specifically to the body, were revealed in stories about addiction and sex. The key question about "moral insight" in 2010 concerned the episode of violence between Kyrgyz and Uzbeks that left everyone shocked. The stories refract and shape reality, but ultimately point beyond "narrated reality," to that which cannot be said, to the "really real" (van de Port 1998).

Awe

"Do you know that [Captain Jacques] Cousteau[23] accepted Islam? [On his sea journeys] he discovered that salt and sweet water do not mix. When he found out that this is exactly how it is written in the Koran, he immediately accepted Islam." Maksat mentioned this during our *dawat*, but he was not the first to tell me the story. Many practicing Muslims in Kyrgyzstan (and in Georgia) had told me about Captain Cousteau's instantaneous conversion on receiving proof of the scientific validity of the Koran. One reason for the captain to be mentioned in conversations was surely because the story of this respectable and famous European (television) scientist might also inspire *me* to convert. Beyond this, the fascination with Cousteau reflected the desire to bolster religious authority with scientific means. (A poignant detail—although irrelevant to the argument—is that Cousteau never publicly confirmed his alleged conversion to Islam and was buried according to the Roman Catholic funerary rites). In similar fashion, newly practicing Muslims in Kyrgyzstan regularly cited the health benefits of regular prayer—as comparable to physical exercise—and talked about participating in Ramadan as a detox of sorts. For Muslims who had lived with the truths of scientific atheism such rationalizations had legitimizing power, meanwhile demonstrating an elective affinity between the teachings of Soviet ethics and Islam (cf. Luehrmann 2011).[24] In this post-atheist environment, the discoveries of a Western television scientist had tremendous appeal.

If in these examples it appeared to be science rather than religion that held supreme authority, then this was only so because the involved *dawatchis* had not yet fully understood (or internalized) the Tablighi message that science is ultimately powerless, as suggested not only by Cousteau's conversion but also the following example. On the second day of *dawat*, Kanat was assigned the task to give the *baian* after the afternoon prayers. He decided to speak about the universe and its perplexing complexity. He was understandably nervous, but told me (and himself) that he shouldn't be because those who deliver a *baian* receive divine assistance. Kanat's speech was a soft-spoken whirlwind of information, in which he took his audience from the tiniest particles—atoms and electrons—to the galaxy of planets and stars. The lecture was effective because of Kanat's calm and trust-inspiring manner of speaking and his known position as a doctor of science, which accentuated his claim that not even scientists understand the workings of the universe, and that they are equally fascinated by the fact that the universe displays such an amazing harmony. "Think about it," he stressed, "everything in this world and beyond is willed by Allah, all is part of His plan."

The references to science resonated with post-Soviet sensibilities and were meant to demonstrate Islam's superiority. Kanat's insistence that scientists are equally baffled by the complexity of the micro- and macro-cosmos and the alleged conversion of television-scientist Cousteau exemplify this. They conform to the following logic: the limitations of science produce awe for the Creation, thereby demonstrating God's omnipotence. This omnipotence manifests itself all around us, visible to those who pay attention, as the following example illustrates.

One afternoon we were seated in the central mosque of Bishkek with six *dawatchis*, listening to the consultations of one of the *alims*. He reached for his smartphone and showed a picture of clouds that formed the name Allah in Arabic. "You see, God makes himself known to us all the time, we just need to pay attention." We spent the next thirty minutes watching a series of videos that demonstrated divine power, including one featuring a girl whose tears turned into crystals, and one of a snake that slithered out of a grave after the funeral had ended. The gathered men clicked their tongues in amazement at these proofs of divine power. An additional example was a video of the central mosque in Mecca at night, when, at a certain point, the entire mosque lit up. The *alim* explained that this was due, not to artificial light, but the energy released by prayer, and he marveled at the possibilities of technology: "Sometimes we are not able to see clearly with our eyes, but the camera will nevertheless record it." The videos produced a momentary awe factor, powerfully evoking divine power. And yet they could easily backfire. One *dawatchi* told me afterward, "There are many fakes among these videos, but it wouldn't have been right for me to challenge the *alim.*"

Desire

The invocation of science and its limitations was attractive, but remained at some distance from everyday concerns, and lacked the kind of emotive energy evident in stories about sex, such as the following one that was shared during one of the *dawats* I took part in: "In paradise I will have a racing car and drive 500,000 kilometers an hour, and I won't even have to fear an accident." Amir Seyit was narrating not his own but his friend's imaginations of paradise, which included one particularly poignant one: "[In paradise] the most beautiful virgins will desire to be with me. So you know what I will do? I will have them play football with each other and I will make love to the ones who score a goal." These fantasies, even in this secondhand rendering, were able to captivate the audience of *dawatchis.* According to Seyit, whenever his friend would tell those stories, even the *aksakals* [Kyrgyz, old men] would all listen attentively.

To be sure, not all fantasies were as promiscuous as this one. During another *dawat, amir* Nur Islam explained to us that in paradise "the heart of your wife will exclaim your name with every beat." This combination of pure devotion and loyalty was particularly attractive because, the *amir* continued, one's wife "will be a thousand times more beautiful in paradise than she is in the world."

It is impossible to determine with certainty the extent to which such stories were accepted as true by the *dawatchi.* Some appeared to take them for the truth, others may have hoped that they were true, or were simply intrigued by the thought of it all. But it was also clear that being on *dawat* intensified their experienced reality. The *dawatchis* were in male-only company where they had to improvise and fend for themselves, that is, where they were able to be men and feel like men. It is in that context that the stories and fantasies were narrated and listened to with a greater level of intensity than they would have been outside the *dawat* context.

An important question is why these stories were so attractive to these men, beyond the possibility that men in general are enticed by prospects of limitless sex and enhanced virility. What was significant was that my acquaintances' experiences compared rather poorly with the presented visions of sex and masculinity. In fact, many of the *dawatchis* in the *jamaat* had difficulties in their relationships with women. Rashid Sultanovich had been kicked out by his wife two years earlier (before he became involved in *dawat*), after which he had lived in a shell of a house at the outskirts of Bishkek without water or heating. My smoking buddy Maksat told me about the throbbing headaches his wife caused in him, and he repeatedly lamented her nagging and constant criticism of his inability to financially provide for his family. *Amir* Seyit, at thirty-two, had never been married and was still living with his mother. He admitted that it was time for him to find a wife, but since he was jobless this was not all that easy. And Kanat commented that *dawat* had complicated his marriage, and he talked about his dream to marry a "real Muslim girl," instead of having an independent wife with her own career.

It is against this background that the significance of stories about women and sex becomes evident. The stories expressed the hope that through *dawat* the men would solve some of their relational and marital problems. Success stories were actively shared, such as the following one: "My wife would always scold me . . . but once I started to go on *dawat* regularly, she became much softer. One time when I returned from *dawat*, I entered the house and she asked me: 'Are you hungry my dear? Just sit down, I will prepare food for you.'" Often, when we were having such conversations one of the experienced *dawatchis* would say that this was all very well, but that ultimately our experiences in this world are insignificant in comparison to the next. As *amir* Seyit put it: "Everyone creates his own heaven, but the real heaven will be much better, it is beyond *any* imagination. When you approach heaven and you see its entrance, you will look at it in awe for forty thousand years."

Justice

In late June 2010, a week after the three-day conflict between Kyrgyz and Uzbeks had left its deadly and destructive traces in southern Kyrgyzstan, people were trying to grasp what had happened. *Dawatchis* in Bishkek were no different. Like others, they wanted to understand why these events were happening. Seated in the mosque, *alim* Muhammad was asked by one of the men gathered there: "How is it possible that this is happening in Kyrgyzstan, given that *dawat* is more active here [than in neighboring countries]?" The question was troubling because it seemed to contradict the shared notion that when you give to Allah, you will receive back manifold. *Alim* Muhammad had his answer ready: "Think of how we relate to children. Imagine that you are watching children at a playground. If someone else's child misbehaves, you won't be concerned; you will think: that's their problem, not mine. But surely you won't be that complacent when one of your own children is misbehaving. You will reprimand and punish them." He paused, looked around as if to make sure that everyone had understood the message, and then added: "There is more to it. You know, the places where *dawat* is strong, those are also the places where Satan tries to fight back."

Judging from the responses, this explanation managed to convince. And yet the logic could be bent in multiple directions. A few days before listening to *alim* Muhammad, I overheard another experienced *dawatchi* (addressed with the title *kudama*) who offered a radically different interpretation. He was talking about Uzgen, a town that was infamous for the eruption of ethnic violence in 1990, but where, contrary to expectations, everything remained calm in 2010 when violence ravaged nearby cities.[25] This miraculous absence of violence, he explained, was because *dawat* had been more active in Uzgen than in other towns in the south. It was proof that Allah protects those who go on *dawat*.

While the *alim* interpreted the violence as reflecting a father punishing his beloved children or because of Satan's countermoves, this other explanation suggested that Allah's children were spared because they had been more active in *dawat*. Because of the flexibility of Tablighi (or other religious) logic, it is a useful vehicle for making crises understandable and digestible. Any event could be interpreted as either gift or punishment by Allah, or alternatively as the work of Satan.[26] Simultaneously, this flexibility also constituted the weakness of the logic, and it was dependent on not asking too many questions. As Seyit put it: "It is wrong to question everything—what counts is how you act, how many *zikrs* (remembrances of God) you say, and how regularly you pray—that's much more important than knowing the answers. Reading *suras* is good, but if you start adding up and comparing all the interpretations, your head starts spinning." For Seyit the response to "heads that are spinning" would be acceptance, which is accomplished during *dawat* and contributes to the intensity of experience. But it is not necessarily of a permanent nature.

The Route Back

After three nights and days the *dawat* fellowships return to their sending mosque. This final part of *dawat* is meant to provide further spiritual food that will sustain the travelers until their next three-day *dawat*, in principle one month later. It is also the moment when inquiries are made about intentions to go on a forty-day *dawat*. On two occasions at which I was present this final "briefing" had an energizing, or at least a consolidating, effect: the travelers narrated how *dawat* had strengthened their relationship with God and how it had provided them with new knowledge. Several of the travelers expressed an intention to go on a forty-day *dawat*, and travelers who had befriended each other agreed on the date for their next three-day *dawat*.

The August *dawat* that has formed the basis of my earlier descriptions, however, had an ending that I had not anticipated. We arrived at the mosque exactly at 4:00 p.m. and sat down on the carpets outside in the open air. The coordinators who debriefed our fellowships asked each of us to reflect on our experiences. The first one to respond was Kanat. He stayed in line with etiquette when commenting that this *dawat* had strengthened his commitment. He mentioned that during the previous three days he had witnessed the power of *dawat*. To sustain this claim he mentioned that after we had made a request (*dua*) for food, the villagers had come out to give us food, and that our prayers for making the *gasht* successful had resulted in several villagers coming to listen to the sermon (*baian*). In response, Kanat received the straightforward advice to improve his regularity in prayer and *dawat*. The next traveler up (named Bolot) echoed this advice by saying that he was still struggling to achieve regularity, and nodded when the coordinator stressed that in comparison to eternity we are asked to sacrifice only a very small amount of time. Several others followed, but then the positive flow was interrupted by Edil, who reported, "I understand everything, but my heart remains closed. It is as if it is blocked. Something just doesn't allow it to change." Perhaps his honesty was unexpected, because the coordinator struggled to give satisfactory advice. The last person to speak said that he was confused more than anything else. While on *dawat* he had felt "something," but now all that remained was ambivalence. Possibly his nonchalant voice provoked the coordinator to emphasize sternly: "It is not that we go on *dawat* for three days and then have the rest of the month off!"

When leaving the mosque Bolot asked if Kanat would lend him money. Knowing Kanat as a generous and economically well-off person, I was surprised that he refused to lend his fellow *dawatchi* the small sum requested. Instead he offered to buy groceries, which Bolot politely declined. Afterward, Kanat explained that Bolot was an alcoholic, and several times had come to *dawat* while still drunk: "When he is on *dawat* it is fine, but in between he loses it." Kanat had asked the elders at the mosque, who advised against lending money, but to try and support him otherwise.

In 2010 I met up again with five of the *dawatchis* I had traveled with the previous year. Edil, who at the time had been struggling with commitment, managed to sideline his doubts. He divorced his wife and married a practicing Muslim from a religious family. *Amir* Nur Islam similarly continued to be actively involved. But for Ruslan, Rashid Sultanowich, and Kanat it was different. Ruslan had stopped going on *dawat*, but emphasized that *dawat* had helped him overcome the chronic backaches that doctors had been unable to cure. Rashid Sultanowich was still involved, but no longer maintained the regularity of the previous year. Kanat had been unable to go on *dawat* for the last four months. He explained that the worldview of the Tablighis had become too restrictive for him:

> As long as you are inside it, it all makes perfect sense, but from the outside it looks differently. There are those who give up their jobs, who lose their families. And to be honest, this started to happen to me too. My job suffered as I spent all my time and energy on *dawat*. And then one day I came home and found my wife crying. It was her birthday, she had bought tickets for the movies, and I had been too busy with *dawat*. That is when I decided to shift my focus. I think that there is a time when you need to be actively involved, and then there is a time when you need to find a balance again.

The logic of the Tablighi method is precisely to ensure that a balance is found between *dawat* and everyday life. But for many *dawatchis* this was difficult to achieve. The *dawat* experience was so intense because the men felt a release from their everyday commitments, and yet this was also why it tended to remain a "bracketed reality." Finding a balance depended on the strength of the Tablighi network as it continued to exist in between the periods of traveling. Such a network was certainly developing, and Kanat often made a point of helping out his acquaintances from *dawat*, for example, by making sure that he bought from their stores. But for the moment, the gap between life among Tablighi brothers and life at home continued to loom large for many of the travelers.

The Pulsation of *Dawat*

The Tablighi Jamaat, like some Christian missions, is acutely aware of the need to provide regular boosts of energy lest people's conviction and devotion dissipate. In the movement's literature this is known as the "dry-dock parable" in which man is compared to a ship that is constantly being rocked by rough waves that damage the ship and steer it off course. In order to deal with these distracting and troubling worldly forces, Muslims need to have regular access to a space of refuge (or dry dock) in the form of the mosque or a *jamaat* (fellowship), where they can be spiritually nourished and replenished.[27]

This pulsating quality of conviction resonated in many stories told by *dawatchis*: Nur Islam compared *dawat* to food, of which the body always desires more. "When you go back to the world, you are faced with constant demands. It is always about money. You find yourself sitting at the table not wanting to listen anymore." It was for this reason, he said, that he avoided speaking about nonreligious topics during *dawat*. The stories also revealed that the distinction between everyday life and life during *dawat* consisted of several dimensions. On the one hand, *dawat* was, as in the parable, a space of refuge from the turmoil of everyday life. Maksat, for example, told me: "You know, this feels like a holiday. Just being here, no problems, no stress." *Dawat* provided relaxation by offering a place of withdrawal from everyday difficulties, and a space to fantasize about different realities. But this experience of relaxation was complemented by an experience of intensification that was rooted in the joint activities of the men and their exposure to the reactions of the villagers (and officials) they encountered en route. This tension between relaxation and intensification generated affective energies from within.[28] Indeed, it was in relation to both these aspects that the constant circulation of stories created an atmosphere in which one was able to come closer to Allah, and in which signs of God's presence became more credible. However, we have seen that the elation can dissipate quickly. As a former *dawatchi* told me: "When you are on *dawat*, everything makes perfect sense. But afterward it appears too simplistic." The logic that is so powerful when part of a fellowship looks different when the social surrounding is made up of people who are not connected to the Tablighis.

The immediate and the longer-lasting effects of the *dawat* experience depended on the temporal and social contexts in which they unfolded, as illustrated by the comments of Kyrgyz and Pakistani *dawatchis* about each other during a joint *dawat*. The differences between them were a frequent topic of conversation, with the Kyrgyz saying that the most significant difference was that the Pakistani had been born and raised in Islam. They admired the Pakistani for their certainty, and stability in matters of faith. And they complained about their own difficulties of having grown up during atheist times and living in a largely secular society. By contrast, the Pakistani expressed amazement about the intensity with which Kyrgyz were able to live their faith, and they repeatedly commented on their fervor and energy.

What we seem to have here, then, are two different modalities of religious experience. For the Pakistani, Islam was part of their habitus, of the world with which they had been familiar since their youth. To them, *dawat* was important to sustain their commitment, and to ensure that their belief (*yiman*) would not turn into indifference. For the Kyrgyz, *dawat* was about something different: it was about overcoming doubt, and hence the cycles of believing and disbelieving were much more intense. Interestingly, this pattern could be observed, not only among individual *dawatchi*, but with reference to the Tablighi movement in Kyrgyzstan more generally. As one Kyrgyz scholar who associates himself with the Tablighi Jamaat told me: "In the 2000s, the number of three-day *jamaats* traveling in the northern regions on weekends was nearing a thousand. This was the period of highest popularity reaching levels of fashion. Since then the numbers have dropped significantly, but [now] there is more regularity, experience, and formalization/legalization of the practice." The trade-off between intensity and regularity, between charisma and routine, are there for everyone to see. The particularities of this trade-off, in a post-Soviet context where Islam returned to the public sphere, help us understand both the power and the fragility of conviction.

5

PENTECOSTAL MIRACLE TRUTH
ON THE FRONTIER

The miracle occurred on a cold Sunday morning in March 2004, in a
poorly lit basement, actually a restaurant, which doubled as church hall
for a chapter of the Church of Jesus Christ.[1] The service had started with
the usual worship songs, but soon everyone's attention rested on one of the
congregants. Venera, a Kyrgyz woman in her twenties, had not spoken a
single word in her life, and was about to be cured of her speech impediment.
The prayers of the approximately seventy congregants waxed and waned,
their sound joined outcries for divine intervention, producing a rhythm
that made the air heavy with anticipation and full of energy. This was the
kind of atmosphere in which one would expect the Holy Spirit to descend.
Pastor Kadyrjan stood right in front of Venera and pressed his hand on her
forehead. The tension in the air was palpable, and anticipation peaked. The
phrase "Help her, Jesus" came from everywhere. Still nothing happened.
Venera stood trembling in the middle. Then, when some started to give up
hope, the Holy Spirit descended on Venera, and she started to speak. She
spoke hesitantly and barely audibly to most congregants, but those who
stood closest reported that the first word she uttered in her life was "Jesus"
(Russian, *Iisus*).

The miracle left me wondering about how to position myself in relation to
the truth of miracles. If I accepted the miracle's divine nature, would that
not indicate I had lost the critical distance deemed indispensable for analysis? But if I denied the possibility of divine intervention, would that not
amount to positivistic reductionism and reveal atheist bias? If the former
were the case, I might marvel at God's inscrutable ways and suggest that
the miracle demonstrated the power of prayer. That view is what Bakyt,
one of the congregants, expressed to me after the service had ended and
we were having lunch in a nearby *chaikhana* (tea house). If, by contrast,

I adopted a secular perspective, then I might analyze how the buildup of momentum produced merely the illusion of a miracle. To prove this point I could have stressed that those who had suggested that Venera called out "Jesus" later mentioned that they were not sure and that perhaps it had only been a grunt. In fact, this is what Bakyt—the same Bakyt—told me a couple of weeks after the events, when it turned out that Venera had not made further progress in learning to speak.

Despite their centrality in Pentecostal churches, miracles have rarely featured as an *analytical* theme in studies of Pentecostalism. This is partly due to the awkwardness of the truth question; so even when the scholarly gaze has rested on miracles, it has tended to evade the issue of truth. Thus, one prominent writer has argued that "analytically there is no observable difference between true and false miracles" (de Vries 2001, 27). Bruce Kapferer, moreover, suggests there is no need to engage with the truth question because the significance of magic and miracles is in their effect and affect (2003, 23–24; see also Ewing 1994). Such approaches rightfully reject positivistic reductionism, but in this rejection they risk excluding more productive engagements with the truth question. That is, by not examining how truth is produced, they leave important analytical opportunities untouched. As Charles Hirschkind argues, attention needs to be paid to how people distinguish between true and false miracles (2011, 94). Indeed, effect and affect cannot be understood without addressing the truth question, especially when the reality of miracles—their truth—is not taken for granted by the involved, as was often the case in Kyrgyzstan. Bakyt's shifting perception regarding the miracle's truthfulness profoundly influenced how he spoke about the event and potentially affected his relationship with the church. This underlines the importance of analyzing the trajectories of miracle truth.

I maintain that a focus on miracles is intellectually productive precisely because the mysterious and unstable qualities of miracles (and their truth) resonate with the unstable nature of conviction. This resonance can be illustrated with reference to the term "charisma." Charisma is a quality of the present, revealed in the here and now, which cannot easily be durably transposed across time or space. Charisma as divine gift is what makes Pentecostalism both effervescent and transient. But understood in a secular Weberian sense, charisma is also the key source of authority "at times of distress," when legal structures have collapsed and tradition has been uprooted, as was the case in post-Soviet Kyrgyzstan.[2] That is, the sociopolitical context in which the miracle occurred was itself unstable.

Pastor Kadyrjan often made comments about the economic and social environment, seeing his church as being involved in a larger battle between the forces of good and evil. He and his wife had moved from Bishkek to Jalalabad in 1999 to "plant" a church branch. It had taken several years of hardship to build a sizable and reasonably stable congregation. The problem at the time was, according to Kadyrjan, that Jalalabad city had been covered in the "spirit of death" (*dukh smerta*). He and his struggling congregation had been thrown out of the venues they had rented several times. But they fought back. Thanks to the collective prayers of his church the city had been (partially) transformed: the "spirit of death" dissolved, resulting in inhabitants becoming more energetic and innovative; there was a decrease in crime, proper shops (rather than market stalls) appeared, and hygiene in the streets improved. Moreover, in early 2004 Kadyrjan was able to purchase a large, if dilapidated, warehouse that was being transformed into a church hall. This was a real victory because it meant the congregation finally had a stable location they could call their own.

In these same four years Kadyrjan had overseen the "planting" of five new congregations in the province. Some of these new congregations were growing steadily, but not the congregation in Kokjangak, which therefore frequently occupied his mind. In fact there had been several attempts to establish a congregation in Kokjangak, but each attempt, he explained, had been sabotaged. His most recent endeavors seemed initially successful when approximately sixty people attended services for several months, but by early 2004 the majority of these attendants stopped coming. Instead of being disillusioned, Kadyrjan was convinced that these difficulties contained an important sign: "It means that [Kokjangak] is under the spell of Satan, and, if that is so, it must mean that Kokjangak is somehow a strategic place." In Kadyrjan's view, the establishment of a vibrant congregation in Kokjangak would deliver a serious blow to Satan's powers, and thereby ease the advance of Christianity in other locations as well. For the time being Kadyrjan instructed Gulbarchyn, whom he had sent to the town as a missionary and local church leader, to intensify the collective praying on top of a hill overlooking Kokjangak in an effort to change the atmosphere in the town.

We may not want to follow Kadyrjan in attributing success and failure to a larger cosmic battle, while still appreciating that the concept of *struggle* shaped and defined this Pentecostal church, and that the effects of this struggle could be counterintuitive. As Pastor Kadyrjan once told me: "We pray for [local government] officials to stop hindering us. But this may not be God's way. Our faith thrives when it is being repressed." For Kadyrjan, it was essential to remain on the offensive and to confront the "dark forces" that surrounded his church. As I will go on to argue, it is this "frontier mentality"[3] that is at the core of the production of conviction. And yet, as we will see, the forward-moving drive eventually reaches its limits, with the forces that produced conviction ultimately responsible for its demise. It is at this intersection that the convergence between conviction and "miracle truth" is clearest. Both are produced on the edge, under the strain of forces that can propel as well as crush them. The truth of miracles becomes simultaneously more pertinent and less stable as we move into the frontier, not least because the "power of prayer" is more difficult to sustain in contexts where success stories are few and congregations are fragile. The unstable Pentecostal mission carried out on the "postatheist" Muslim-Christian frontier offers a stark illustration of the effervescent as well as fragile qualities of Pentecostal conviction.

The Post-Soviet Pentecostal Frontier

With approximately forty thousand church members in 2004, the success of Evangelical-Pentecostal Christianity in post-Soviet Kyrgyzstan has been remarkable. This is not to say that Pentecostal Christianity was completely new to the region. In Soviet Kyrgyzstan several underground Pentecostal churches had been active, including one in Kokjangak, but my Kyrgyz Pentecostal acquaintances referred to these somewhat dismissively as "traditional" and "legalistic," which anyway only catered to a narrow circle of Russians. It was only after the collapse of the USSR that Pentecostal churches started to attract larger numbers, including people of Muslim background. By 2004 approximately twenty-five thousand Kyrgyz had converted to Evangelical-Pentecostal Christianity (ethnic Kyrgyz made up approximately 60 percent of these churches, alongside Russians, Koreans, Tatars, and others). Boasting ten thousand tithe-paying members and forty-five congregations throughout Kyrgyzstan, the Church of Jesus Christ was the largest Evangelical-Pentecostal Church in the country.

This section discusses the advance of the Church of Jesus Christ and asks how Pentecostalism, with its characteristics of rupture, charisma, and intensity, resonated with the post-Soviet Muslim geography in which it advanced. Given that conversion from Islam to Christianity is exceptional and rare, it is relevant to ask how and why conversion became an option for some Kyrgyz, that is, how the conditions that made conversion possible had emerged historically. This is particularly significant because in the pre-Soviet period the idea of conversion to Christianity was inconceivable to the Kyrgyz. Missionary activities, such as those of German Mennonites in Talas Province in the first decade of the twentieth century, had instead reinforced the notion that Christianity was a religion of alien Europeans and that Kyrgyz were Muslim by definition (Pelkmans 2009a, 3–4). However, seventy years of antireligious campaigning and Soviet modernization profoundly altered the playing field.

From the late 1920s onward, Soviet antireligious policies destroyed Islamic institutions, curtailed the circulation of religious knowledge, and "domesticated" Islamic practices (see Khalid 2006 for a good discussion). This did not mean that Islam was completely eradicated. Ironically, in fact, Soviet rule affirmed the connection of ethnic and religious identities. The implicit contradiction in the Soviet attempt to repress religion while promoting culture, when in fact the two cannot be easily disentangled, resulted in the incorporation of many "religious" practices into a standardized "cultural" or Kyrgyz repertoire. This also meant that adherence to an ethno-national group automatically conjured up a specific religious tradition. Even when not professed, religion continued to be a key marker of difference. Thus, Kyrgyz members of the Communist Party, even those who held an atheist worldview, would still claim to be Muslims, as this indicated their cultural background. Indeed, as we saw in chapter 3, the notion of "atheist Muslim" was not perceived as an oxymoron. The resulting "cultural Islam" was largely devoid of Islamic knowledge and religious effervescence, and therefore vulnerable to subsequent post-Soviet challenges.

Such "national" forms of religion flourished in the initial phases of the post-Soviet period. But the "nationalization" of religion also produced discontent from within, and excluded those who fell outside the bounds of the (imagined) nation. In addition, "nationalized" religions became increasingly vulnerable when, as in the case of Kyrgyzstan, the newly independent states failed to deliver on promises of affluence, stability, and security. These tensions between national and religious categories produced various outcomes. Discontent with "official" Islamic structures reinforced the attractiveness of decentralized Islamic networks such as those of the Tablighi Jamaat that voiced frustration with the outcome of postsocialist "transition" and offered their own versions of "true Islam." However, as we saw in the previous chapter, the views of such new Muslim movements were not always compatible with the ideas of post-Soviet citizens, especially those of urban women. The tensions thus produced rendered these women's original Muslim identity increasingly problematic, creating a space in which many women—especially those in marginal positions—felt drawn to Evangelical and Pentecostal communities.

In short, Soviet secularism had relegated religious expression to the domestic sphere while contributing to the objectification of religion, which enabled Kyrgyz actors to consider their position vis-à-vis Islam. This condition of possibility coincided with the Kyrgyz government adopting the most liberal religious policies of all post-Soviet Central Asian countries, which in practice meant that missions and churches faced few state-imposed obstacles (in the period between 1991 and 2008). The destabilization of Islam and the liberal policies of the Kyrgyz government created an environment in which Evangelical-Pentecostal churches could be active and relatively successful. Although this background sketch suggests why conversion was conceivable, we now need to look at the appeal of Pentecostalism in the post-Soviet context.

The attractiveness of Evangelical-Pentecostal churches was partly constituted through the general appeal that the West had in the wake of the Soviet collapse. They represented "the modern," understood here as the promise "to reorder society by applying strategies that have produced wealth, power, or knowledge elsewhere in the world" (Donham 1999, xviii). But while the association with the "modern West" proved advantageous to the position of Pentecostalism, it is important to note that the most successful churches in Kyrgyzstan were not foreign missionary churches but rather those run by Kyrgyzstani citizens of various ethnic backgrounds (see Wanner 2007 for a similar observation regarding Ukraine). The Church of Jesus Christ is a case in point. It boasted its connections to international Christian networks such as Calvary International, the Russian Union of Christians of Evangelical Faith, and Derek Prince International. But the church was not founded or run by foreign missionaries. Ever since its foundation in the early 1990s it had been led by local pastors, with the senior pastor being an ethnic Russian (born in Kyrgyzstan), and Pastor Kadyrjan in Jalalabad (like most pastors outside the capital) an ethnic Kyrgyz. The combination of transnational involvement and local organization allowed the church to present a transnational image and to muster international support when necessary, while its home-grown leadership ensured that it was plugged into the realities of Kyrgyzstani society.

The Church of Jesus Christ grew rapidly. In the mid-1990s it "planted" church branches in the major cities and some district centers in the north; around the turn of the millennium the church expanded its activities in the south of the country. This implied a move from a region with a strong Russian presence and that was locally seen as secularized to a region that was seen as more Islamic. As mentioned above, Pastor Kadyrjan established his congregation in Jalalabad 1999, and over the next four years oversaw the planting of five additional branches in the Jalalabad region. These geographical shifts were paralleled by changes in the ethnic makeup of the congregations. While in Bishkek a (slight) majority of church members was Russian, in Jalalabad 75 percent of the approximately two hundred tithe-paying members were Kyrgyz.

Important aspects of the church's attractiveness and success were its organization and message. The church offered not only salvation, but access to prosperity, health, and success by faithful prayer. Moreover, it did so by integrating its members into a tightly organized community of "believers." Apart from the weekly service, all members were expected to take part in "home-church" meetings (*domashnaia tserkov'*) that would gather at least once a week. During home-church meetings, the congregants collectively pray, study the Bible, discuss their efforts in combating addictions and poverty, and testify about the ways in which God changes their lives, thus reinforcing the church's theology in an intimate setting.

It is easy to see the attractions of this Pentecostal message and organization to people living in a state of "post-Soviet chaos" (Nazpary 2002), who are struggling with the effects of an unraveling welfare state in which life became more difficult and less predictable, especially for those who found themselves at the margins of society. These factors were reflected in the overrepresentation of marginalized groups in the church's demography. The Jalalabad congregation consisted of 75 percent women, slightly more than half of whom had lost a husband through divorce or death. Moreover, the vast majority of church members (71%) were migrants to the city, the majority of which had migrated there after the Soviet collapse (based on a survey among 121 congregants; see Pelkmans 2009b, 152–53 for details). Although I cannot provide percentages, it was quite common for congregants to have suffered from addictions before they came to the church.

The church acknowledged such patterns, and in the capital proactively engaged with it, for example, through its elaborate outreach programs to prisoners and the homeless. When asked, church representatives explained overrepresentation of marginalized people with reference to Jesus's teaching that "the last will be first and the first will be last" (Matt. 20:16). Pentecostalism offers hope and direction to shattered lives, and concrete answers for dealing with the multifaceted existential uncertainty of post-Soviet life. Moreover, the idea that divine intervention can be invoked by prayer pushes people to assert their agency in dealing with an unruly world, that is, to tame the unpredictable forces of the post-Soviet chaos (see also Wanner 2007).

As is typical for Pentecostal conversion, church members reported an experience of radical discontinuity (cf. Robbins 2007). They presented their conversion as having plunged into their new belief, pushing aside hesitations and apparently overcoming their initial confusion.[4] But these radical conversions were not necessarily of a permanent nature. Possibly because the speed of conversion meant that their worries and confusions were never fully resolved, possibly also because life in the late Soviet period had taught people to be reticent about official proclamations of truth, it meant that these new truths did not always become permanently internalized and that their suppressed doubts could easily resurface. The destabilization of fields of meaning and practice created an environment in which everything was potentially true and possibly a lie, which also meant that new religions were not always very firmly, or very permanently, embraced. Two kinds of uncertainty converge here: epistemological uncertainty (referring to knowledge) and existential uncertainty (referring to conditions of life). The centrality of miracles reflects this uncertainty, both in the sense that miracles work to overcome such existential uncertainty and in the sense that their epistemological status remained unstable.

Producing Pentecostal Truth

Zamira had moved to Jalalabad city a couple of years before we met in the autumn of 2003. Her marriage had ended, which meant that she had had to leave her in-laws' village home and move with her two daughters to the city. She was lucky to find a new job as a teacher, but surviving on an inadequate salary in a city where she had no direct relatives was an uphill battle. The battle became an imminent crisis when her five-year-old daughter fell seriously ill.

> I didn't have any options left. I had taken my daughter everywhere—to the mullah [here: Islamic healer], the hospital—but all they did was take my money. That's when I accepted [my colleague's] offer to take me to her church. For a whole night I didn't sleep; I stayed up and prayed. I gave myself over to God, asked Jesus for forgiveness. And by the next day my daughter started to feel better!

Zamira joined the church's home group meetings straightaway, meanwhile keeping her conversion hidden from her relatives. When they found out several months later, they were shocked. Her brothers, one of whom had been involved in an Islamic piety movement, accused her not only of apostasy but also of betraying her Kyrgyz-ness (*kyrgyzchylyk*). Her parents also responded negatively, but they increasingly "took it for what it was. They knew how I had suffered from the sickness of my daughter," Zamira said. She stressed that since then she had continuously witnessed to others "about the healing of my daughter through Jesus Christ, and that He has completely transformed my life. I have witnessed to my acquaintances, my relatives, my colleagues."

This story is one of many that I collected among members of the Church of Jesus Christ, in Bishkek, Jalalabad, and Kokjangak. Zamira's account has many parallels with Pentecostal conversion stories from other parts of the world. The swiftness of conversion, the discourse of discontinuity (Meyer 1998; Robbins 2007), and the importance of witnessing (Coleman 2003) are elements that feature prominently in Pentecostal discourse and practice worldwide. As one would expect to be the case in any Muslim context, Zamira's conversion to Christianity was controversial and drew hostile responses from relatives, but Zamira's actions also illustrate how seventy years of Soviet antireligious modernization had eroded the position of Islam to the extent that conversion was a distinct possibility.

The central feature in the story, however, was healing through divine intervention. Numerous converts told me that they first became interested in the Church of Jesus Christ after hearing of the healing powers ascribed to Pastor Kadyrjan. As in the case of Zamira, who came into contact with the church during her search for medical aid, many approached the church with the hope of being cured of illness or addiction. And like Zamira, they often had previously visited the hospital or local spiritual healers or both, without obtaining the desired effect. As one male congregant said, "I thought that they [Kadyrjan and his wife] were a kind of shaman [Kyrgyz, *shamandar*], especially when I heard them speak in tongues" during a service. Healing was not just the point of first contact, but an important element in conversion experiences. A former alcoholic mentioned that one night she went into the street and cried out: "Jesus, if you are the living God, please help me." After that, she collapsed, later waking up in the house of a church leader, having lost the desire to drink alcohol. Another common theme was how God helped combat poverty. Almaz, a young man, told me, "For a long time I didn't have work. Then, on January 19, 2004, I prayed to God and asked for work. The following day, when I was having lunch in town, I was invited to work. I understood that God had heard me."

As will have become clear, my acquaintances in the church saw evidence of divine power in many corners of life. It was detected in the slow and creeping changes in the cityscape as suggested by Pastor Kadyrjan in the introduction of this chapter, and was just as likely to be witnessed in fleeting events, as when during a service the worship leader ascribed the return of electricity (after a power outage that had lasted for an hour) to the Holy Spirit. Divine power was seen to be at work when people recovered from their illnesses, got rid of other physical problems, or were liberated from their addictions. It was evident when they received unexpected help from a neighbor, enjoyed an economic windfall, or received a job after praying, as Almaz experienced.

An important aspect of these examples of divine intervention is their narration. It is through their circulation that happenings may gain status as miracles. To put it differently, central to the miracle business was the process by which people become cognizant of them, and start to recognize miracles in their own lives and in the world around them. Indeed, the church actively encouraged interpreting positive events as gifts of God and as examples demonstrating the effectiveness of prayer. In services and home-church meetings, new converts learned—often literally—to interpret their experiences in terms of Pentecostal thought.

For a happening to *be* a miracle, the decisive factor is that it is caused by divine intervention. But for such a happening to be *recognized* and *acknowledged* as having been caused by divine intervention, several ingredients need to be present. First of all, of course, there needs to be a *favorable* outcome: an addicted person who is liberated, an ill person recovered, a jobless person who receives a job, or indeed an electricity outage that is restored. Second, this outcome should be *unexpected*: the addicted person had tried many times to quit drinking; medical doctors had given up hope of recovery; the jobless person had been jobless for a long time; the electricity returned at exactly the right moment. Two additional features are not indispensable but are conducive to miracle status: the absence of an alternative explanation, and the happening having occurred after (i.e., in response to) the prayers of congregants. Certain phenomena fit these criteria better than others, but the fit is always dependent on interpretation, influenced by presentation, and open to contestation.

The specificities of miracle truth production in the Church of Jesus Christ can be illustrated by a brief contrast with the institutionalized process of miracle validation in the Roman Catholic Church. There, putative miracles are painstakingly documented and registered, examined by experts belonging to a "college of physicians," and tested against the alternative explanations of an official "devil's advocate," before the validity of the miracle can be (hesitantly) acknowledged (Duffin 2007). By contrast miracles were never formally tested in the Church of Jesus Christ. Instead there were powerful informal mechanisms by which miracle truth was produced and generalized. The reality of miracles was affirmed in sermons, shared and communicated informally between congregants, and staged in public encounters.

There was clearly no deficit of miracles in the Church of Jesus Christ. A seemingly paradoxical way of phrasing this would be to say that the miraculous was rather mundane—in the sense that the occurrence of miracles was routine and commonplace. Such an attitude was encouraged within the church. Sermons often focused on the occurrence of miracles, and congregants were encouraged to share their own experiences with divine intervention. Stories of healing through prayer also filled its newspaper *Tvoi Put'* (Russian, *Your Way*) and was a recurring theme in the book series published by the church, seen in titles like *Power in the Name Jesus Christ*, *Breaking the Chains of Slavery*, and *Lord, Help Us to Pray*. The pastors often referred to the power of prayer and the need for committed prayer. Miracles were not to be questioned or scrutinized, but rather repeated and embellished.

Acceptance of miracle truth was facilitated by the links with existing cultural repertoires, and the flexible adjustment to local realities. For example, the senior pastor Kuzin in Bishkek would regularly invoke the dangers of immorality in the city and talk about the spirit of slavery (Russian, *dukh rabstva*) as evident in alcoholism and drug addiction, but I never heard him preach about the evil residing in local forms of spiritual healing. By contrast, in Jalalabad and Kokjangak, references to "occultism" (*okkul'tizm*) were common, as in the following excerpt from a sermon by Pastor Kadyrjan. The preceding week he had been invited to the house of an ailing Kyrgyz girl in Kokjangak. He immediately felt "the ice-cold atmosphere" that indicated the presence of evil. He explained:

> There were pieces of paper with Arabic phrases everywhere: above the door, on the wall, next to her bed. Such a piece of paper floated even in her water jug. The girl had received medicine and had been treated by a *közü-achyk* [Kyrgyz, clairvoyant] and a *moldo* [mullah], but nothing had helped. . . . She feared that if she closed her eyes she would die instantly. Then I told her about Jesus. She didn't understand at first. But when I started to pray, she started to understand, and protested that she was a Muslim. Nevertheless, she agreed to talk about [faith] and she started to feel better. Later I took her out of the house into the sun and she really felt better. When I left she asked me if I could visit her again. I promised her that I definitely would! Praise the Lord!

Following Kadyrjan's example, the local church leader in Kokjangak, Gulbarchyn, tried to identify the evil spirits present in Kokjangak. In her analysis the main types of evil were "witchcraft" or "sorcery" (Russian, *koldovstvo*), the "spirit of destruction" (*dukh razrusheniia*), and the "spirit of poverty" (*dukh nishchety*). But she was open to suggestions that would improve her analysis. She explained that she asked all visiting "believers" about their opinion concerning the evil spirits that needed to be confronted and defeated.

This vocabulary demonstrated the manner in which the church adjusted to different contexts to address locally relevant problems. In fact, there were remarkable similarities between the worldview promoted by Pentecostal churches and local notions about spirits, as well as between Pentecostal faith healing and traditional "Muslim" healing. Kadyrjan once inadvertently commented on this when recollecting that he and his wife had initially often been mistaken for *közü-achyklar* (Kyrgyz, clairvoyants). Or as one of the congregants who had previously been active as a (Muslim) spiritual healer told me: "I saw many miracles of Jesus. I believe that he is savior and healer because when I put my hands with the name of Jesus on ill people they recover." At least two messages can be taken away from these examples: they demonstrated the insistence on adjusting church doctrine to local realities thereby ensuring relevance, and they took seriously previously existing ideas about the spiritual world (see also chapter 6). In contrast to atheist activists and Tablighi Muslims, Pentecostal church leaders did not dismiss "occultism" or "shamanism" as ineffective superstition, but rather incorporated these practices and ideas into their theories of spiritual warfare.

Ideas about miracles, propagated in sermons, made meaningful through their semiotic connections, achieved realness in the *domashka* (Russian, home church). Here, congregants exchange ideas and experiences, and thereby become experienced in recognizing divine influence on events in their lives. Or that's what supposedly happens according to stories told by congregants. They referred to the *domashka* as a space of learning, where the confusing and mysterious aspects of the Pentecostal emphasis on the Holy Spirit became meaningful and understandable. A woman told one such story: "My husband accompanied me to the *domashka* at the pastor's house. The atmosphere was cozy, everyone was uninhibited. They treated me as if they had known me for a long time. Then the pastor and his wife prayed for me. . . . I accepted [Jesus] in my heart, and that same day I was blessed with the Holy Spirit." But it was not just about recognizing God's ways. Inclusion in the *domashka* often facilitated positive transformations in people's lives, also because it provided the mutual support necessary to overcome addictions or to deal with social and economic problems. Zamira commented extensively on this point:

> How shall I put it? The quality of interaction is different. When you meet new people outside [the church] you always need to be cautious. They have their interests, want something from you. They may steer you in the wrong direction. But among believers it is not like that. We call each other brother and sister. And it really feels like that. We watch over each other, help each other not to go the wrong path. During our meetings I feel energized. It feels like, "Yeah, I'm ready for this life."

The surge of Pentecostalism across the post-Soviet landscape resembles in some ways the proliferation of magic. As Galina Lindquist has argued: "Magic deals with uncertainty, . . . neutralizing its destructive potential, and making hope, as a mode of existential orientation, once again possible" (2006, 21). Like magic, Pentecostalism is able to provide direction to agentive power within contexts that are uncertain and appear chaotic.[5] An important difference, though, is that it does so not in a dialogue between two individuals (healer and client) but while embedding people in new solidarity networks. Moreover, these networks are not only about support and guidance, but about jointly facing a hostile external world.

The miracles presented in sermons and embellished in more informal settings had the potential to transform lives: incurable diseases could be cured, long-term addictions overcome, personal flaws repaired, jobs provided. For this potential to be realized, miracles need to be *recognized* as miracles. This point implies that they need to be seen as not only positive and relevant but also meaningful. They need to be, on the one hand, "miraculous," while on the other, believable. There are several tensions at work here. First, miracles were craved most when and where they were least likely to occur. Second, while the church's mundane approach to miracles allowed them to play a central role in everyday life, it also meant that miracles could easily lose their enchantment.

Truth Decay

I asked Aikan if she had experienced any doubts when she became involved with the church three years previously in 2001: "No, not at all!

With me it was rather the other way around. I was proud to be a believer, to go to this church. . . . I didn't doubt anything. I simply—well, I quickly adopted that belief." Not only in this instance but also on other occasions Aikan described her conversion as straightforward and complete. She and her husband had been living in Jalalabad at the time, and like so many others, she had converted through healing. After having visited *bakshis* (Kyrgyz, shamans) without any positive result, her son had been healed by Pastor Kadyrjan. She became an active congregant immediately after her conversion, went out on evangelization trips, and was convinced that her prayers had not only cured her son but also given her a job. Aikan insisted that the church even had a positive influence on her marriage, because after his conversion her husband started to take his role as provider more seriously.

> I liked it when they said that at home the husband needs to command, that the husband should be the one who works, and that women should be able to ask their husbands for household money. . . . When my husband forbade me to go, I told him: "What they say over there is good. They say that at home the husband should be in command, whereas with us it is usually me who scolds you." So then he agreed that I would attend church, and a few months later he also started to go. After that, we both had well-paying jobs and we had a lot of money.

Two years later, for reasons not entirely clear to me, Aikan's husband moved to Bishkek, leaving his wife and children behind. Because they had been living in an apartment that belonged to his relatives, Aikan returned to her native Kokjangak in 2003. After getting by on poor-paying temporary jobs, she began praying fervently for a real job. "I prayed for a job that could be combined with taking care of my children. And then I was given [a job at the city administration]. I didn't search for it; they just came to me and offered me the job." What struck me, however, was that she spoke of this fulfilled wish without emotion, which indicated that she did not perceive it (any longer?) as a miracle. Given the harsh realities of life, this was not so surprising. Her salary was barely sufficient to buy flour, potatoes, and cabbage for herself and her three children. Perhaps it was also because her prayers did not deliver her most intense wish. Aikan had prayed often and intensely for her husband to return.

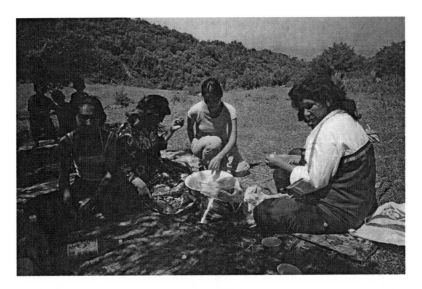

Aikan (second from right) and some of her friends on a picnic in the hills outside Kokjangak, May 2004

Finally, after two years, he visited her house: "He stayed here for fifteen minutes, and then left again, saying he had to go back to Bishkek the very same night."

In the months thereafter Aikan became more irregular in her church attendance, no longer participated in evangelization, and failed to contribute the tithe (church contribution) for several months. Pastor Kadyrjan admonished her to return to the church, but judging from Aikan's words this was unlikely to happen. "I am still interested, that is not the thing. Simply, how can I tell you? I am simply tired of this life. I find it interesting when they talk about God. . . . As long as they sit in my house [during home-church meetings], I listen intensely and then I think 'I should probably do as before.' But it doesn't work out. And I can't pull myself together."

When Aikan described to me the first years of her involvement in the church, she sketched a life of being on a high, an emotional intensity that was somewhat reminiscent of what Venera must have experienced when congregants collectively prayed to cure her speech impediment: a trembling pressure with a clear focal point that produced a momentary outburst of energy. What both stories indicate is that although the church's mechanisms for generating miracle truth were effective in the short term, they faced difficulties in the long run. The example of Venera, who after two weeks was still unable to produce more than just a few sounds (and had she not been able to do that before anyway?), showed that miracles may stop being seen as miraculous. Meanwhile, Aikan's story illustrated that miracles involving healing or employment may lose their gloss or may even cease to be seen as miraculous.

The problem can be referred to as the "charisma paradox." While essential for generating temporary conviction, charisma is inherently unstable. The amazement, the temporary fascination will necessarily wear off. If the charisma is not to evaporate completely, either new miracles need to occur or the charismatic needs to be connected to more permanent structures (i.e., institutionalization).[6] But in neither case will charisma remain what it used to be in the beginning. Whereas new miracles will produce problems of credibility, more permanent structures are likely to result in a loss of effervescence. Aikan's story is illuminating not only because it offers an example of this charisma paradox, but also because it shows that this paradox needs to be understood in relation to the socioeconomic environment in which the miraculous is asserted.

It is decidedly more than a coincidence that Aikan maintained her religious fervor while living in Jalalabad, only to lose it relatively soon after moving back to Kokjangak. In fact, her experiences dovetailed with the trajectories of the Pentecostal congregations in these two locations. As mentioned previously, after a few difficult years the church in Jalalabad began to flourish, boasting 250 tithe-paying members in 2004, most of whom had been with the church for over a year. Although the congregation in Jalalabad certainly fluctuated, the ups and downs were far less dramatic than they were in Kokjangak. When Kadyrjan first started activities there in 2001, he cooperated with locally residing Russian Pentecostals. After attracting a sizable crowd of sixty to eighty Russian and Kyrgyz attendants for a few months, the congregation shrank considerably amid internal bickering. Kadyrjan made a second attempt in fall 2002, when he sent Gulbarchyn, a female Kyrgyz church member, to live as a missionary and church leader in Kokjangak. This time the prospects seemed promising, and for about a year the church services and prayer meetings were well attended, mostly by Kyrgyz women. But by spring 2004 interest had dwindled, and Kadyrjan was worried that his efforts would once again fail to produce the desired results.

On the face of it, Kokjangak would appear to be the perfect environment for the "prosperity gospel." Not only were living conditions miserable, inhabitants believed that a better life should be possible. They had experienced better in the past, and the neoliberal "gospel" trumpeted by the Akaev government (1991–2005) had promised the "second coming" of an earthly paradise. Personally, I had experienced how a (temporary) surge of hope and anticipation was generated when a UNDP development project announced the start of its poverty alleviation program (see chapter 2). The Pentecostal Church, with its promise that earthly success and health were attainable through faithful prayer, was perfectly placed to stimulate the same needs and desires. Indeed, the quick surge of church attendance experienced by the Church of Jesus Christ testified to that very fact.

Pastor Kadyrjan remembered how in the early weeks dozens of people had been baptized in Kokjanagak: "People just came forward by themselves, pushed along by the Spirit." The skeptic might argue that many of these conversions were about experimentation rather than full commitment, but in any case a core was formed of twenty to thirty women (and a few men), who became deeply involved with the church in 2003. But even among them, many ended up being disappointed when the promised prosperity and health failed to arrive. Congregants prayed for an end to poverty, for new jobs, and for success in small business. Although Kadyrjan and other church leaders stressed that the reason their prayers remained unanswered was a lack of faith or lack of devotion in prayer, this type of explanation worked only to a degree. Ultimately, the credibility of prosperity teaching depended on the perceived success of prayer, and the failure to deliver tangible results was therefore a problem that could lead to disillusionment.[7]

Aikan's experiences are particularly instructive in this regard. She had been an experienced church member when she moved to Kokjangak, and was expected to uphold the church view on failure. Church members would argue with her, saying that "if God is alive, then Kokjangak wouldn't have fallen apart and people wouldn't live in such poverty." Aikan's reply to such comments had been that "only the old things are being taken apart. After this, everything will be built up again—and better than before." The question was, however, to what extent she continued to believe these things herself. One evening she told me: "Sometimes I sit by myself and I think, 'What has God given me?' OK, he gave me an apartment, he gave me work, but I prayed for my husband for so long. And what happened? He came and said, 'No, I won't live with you.' So where did my prayers go to then?"

The problem of disillusionment was more pronounced in Kokjangak than it was in Jalalabad. The destitute condition in the former mining town, the lack of stable jobs, and the risk and low pay of others, meant that economic success was a rare exception. Moreover, the patterns of migration and the abundant alcoholism meant that prayers for stable family life and reliable husbands were unlikely to be fulfilled, as Aikan's story illustrated. Even though life in Jalalabad was also hard, its more vibrant economy made success stories more common. Many of the Jalalabad congregants were recent rural-urban migrants who had felt lost in the city and struggled to survive, but once plugged into the congregation's close-knit network, they quite conceivably would find their way upward.

Although conversion to Pentecostalism can be seen as an emancipatory strategy for those involved, the act of conversion complicates relations with the wider society. In the mentioned survey of 121 congregants, more than 60 percent of Kyrgyz respondents reported negative reactions to their conversion, including heated arguments, prohibitions (by parents, husbands, and brothers) on visiting the church again, and (temporarily) deteriorating relations with relatives. Another 10 percent characterized reactions as very negative, including violence, expulsion from home or the family circle, and prolonged attempts at bringing them back to Islam.[8] As the percentages suggest, these challenges were very common, but their effects were far from straightforward. They could both contribute to and detract from commitment to the church.

Ainura, who lived in Jalalabad and was part of a vibrant congregation, told me that her relatives, especially those on her husband's side, had strongly disapproved of her conversion: "They told him to divorce me, they called him to the mosque, and an *ajy* [woman knowledgeable in

Islam] visited me, but I told her that I wouldn't leave God." In fact, the agitation with which she told me her story suggested that these challenges had strengthened her in her faith. Aikan's recollections of her time in Jalalabad were similar. She did have ample negative encounters with "nonbelievers." People used to ask, for example, if they had orgies on special Sundays (replaying Soviet propaganda about the Baptists) and how much she was being paid to show up at the church. Reactions were also often negative on evangelization trips, with people calling her "a traitor" and blaming her for having "sold her religion." But when she lived in Jalalabad these negative encounters failed to erode her faith. As a counterbalance to such negative reactions, there was the church and a relatively large community of "believers" on whom she could lean.

This balance was disrupted after she moved back to Kokjangak. For one, the negative confrontations became more direct, and they were no longer restricted to encounters during evangelization activities. Several times Muslim men came to Aikan's door in the apartment building. Although she insisted that she did not care about such visits, and gave detailed reports of how she replied to their accusations, she still said that one of the hardest things about living in Kokjangak was that everyone knew her as a Christian. On top of the negative reactions she had to face, it turned out that an increasing number of people in her immediate surroundings turned their backs on the Church of Jesus Christ. Home-church meetings that were held in Aikan's apartment used to be well attended, but more and more people "became afraid and stayed away. The *moldo* [mullah] had visited them, or their parents did not agree." Likewise, her brother, who had converted not long after Aikan, visited her one day and said: "Aikan, it turns out that it is a Russian God and not our God. Ugh! I won't go there anymore."

In Jalalabad city negative encounters did not necessarily have a negative impact on the church's prospects. On the contrary, such encounters confirmed the ideas of church members about the corrupt nature of Kyrgyz society and as such increased the cohesiveness of the church. Moreover, negative reactions provided valuable material for testimonies, thus adding to the heroism of "true believers." Another reason why this invigorating dimension existed in Jalalabad was that the church offered a space of refuge for congregants, often rural-urban migrants, who struggled to get by in the relatively anonymous space of the city. In Kokjangak, however, there were far fewer possibilities for retreat. Inhabitants, including members of the church, were in contact with their relatives on a daily basis and depended more heavily on the (non-Christian) social networks that had formed over their lifetime. As such, it appeared that any further growth of the Church of Jesus Christ hinged on both the emergence of a socioeconomic environment that would lend credence to the "power of prayer," and on the stability of the congregation such that it could serve as a viable alternative community capable of neutralizing the hostile reactions of Islamic leaders and others.

By analyzing the relationship between the ideas of the Church of Jesus Christ and the social fabric within which they obtained their experiential reality, we begin to understand the complex dynamics of (temporary) conviction. These dynamics were influenced by the ideology and structure of the church, the motivations and actions of its members, and the responses from (predominantly) Muslim relatives, neighbors, and community leaders. This set of conditions led not only to the creation of Christian niches in a predominantly Muslim environment, but also to the appearance of new dynamics of inclusion and exclusion, which in turn influenced conversion trajectories.

The attraction of Pentecostalism was linked to the destabilization of Muslim and socialist contexts, but its prolonged impact depended on the possibility of demonstrating the fruits of prayer through the achievements of its members, and was thus interrelated with the socioeconomic dynamics of the locality in which it operated. The ethnographic materials contained in this chapter show that the popular idea that the messages of Pentecostalism thrive on social, economic, and political collapse risks ignoring that Pentecostalism needs an environment that offers (at least limited) social and economic opportunities to its members. In other words, the sustainability of new communities of faith also depended on the extent to which the church's promises—of health and wealth—continued to be convincing. This was contingent both on the strength of the congregation within which success stories circulated and on actual possibilities of success. While economic destitution quite straightforwardly limited the reach of the prosperity gospel, the negative responses triggered by the Pentecostal presence in a Muslim-majority situation had more unpredictable results. In the case of Aikan, once the enthusiasm wore off and the experienced miracles lost their gloss, the confrontation with Muslim neighbors resulted in gradual disengagement from the church. But the confrontation with disapproving neighbors and relatives could just as well have the opposite effect, such as in the case of Zamira, contributing to a sense of being uniquely chosen.

It is impossible to establish exactly whether these different outcomes were the result of personal characteristics, the deliverance of the fruits of prayer, or the strength of the congregations. But what is clear is that the dynamics of inclusion and exclusion can contribute to, as well as erode, the structures of faith. As was mentioned in the introduction to this chapter, Pentecostal effervescence needed challenges to produce a sense of exclusivity, of belonging to a chosen group. However, when such external challenges worked on an already weakened congregational structure and when prayer failed to produce success stories, they could easily lead to the erosion of conviction, and to disengagement from the church.

Permanent Struggle

> [Church membership in Jalalabad city] rose to 250 and then it fell again, then it rose again, it is a process we go through. If you would add up all the people who converted in our church, you would probably get to eight hundred people. It happens all the time. People join the church, and then suddenly they say that they no longer have time. And that's the end of it. What happens is that the "open" people come to our church, but then relatives and others start to put pressure on this person, trying to convince them that they should not go to the church, offer money so that they won't go, and if that doesn't help, they will ostracize them. It is the usual thing; persecution is part of Christianity. We pray for [local government] officials to stop hindering us. But this may not be God's way. Our faith thrives when it is being repressed.
>
> PASTOR KADYRJAN

Engaging with the question of miracle truth does not necessarily lead to either positivistic reductionism or a collapse of critical distance. Rather, by taking seriously the empirical observation that miracle truth is unstable, and by analyzing how truth status is ascribed to and removed from specific incidents, important aspects of the working of Pentecostal conviction are revealed.

With its emphasis on prayer and divine intervention, Pentecostalism encountered fertile ground in Kyrgyzstan. The dislocation of society, and the unraveling of the welfare state, produced an environment receptive to

Pentecostal promises. But it was also an unstable one. This instability was reflected in the miracle business. Miracle status was fragile partly because of the unstable characteristics of the post-Soviet condition, highlighting the way in which truth is often less about evidence than about the organization of information (cf. Hastrup 2004, 456). The specific manner in which this information was organized, and how it related to the wider social field, made miraculous happenings momentarily convincing. However, the invocation of the divine could fail to deliver results, and miraculous happenings could lose their charismatic gloss or run up against rival interpretations. The congregants' assessment of miracles depended not only on their epistemological underpinnings but also on the social relations that surrounded these miracles. The encouragement, repetition, and explication of unexpected happenings enabled the production of effervescence. But when these social relations would break down, and on top of this a non-Pentecostal network asserted itself, the truth of miracles started to unravel. The risk of failure was largest in contexts where the need for miracles was greatest, because these were also the situations in which it was most difficult to produce success in the form of jobs, regained health, and reliable husbands. And when effervescence decreased, when doubt set in, the challenge posed by rival epistemological and existential points of reference loomed particularly large. Such processes not only underlined the effervescence of Pentecostal truth, but also highlighted the tension between Pentecostal Christianity and Islam, and the active steps undertaken by relatives and neighbors to dissuade Kyrgyz congregants from engagement with the church.

What needs to be stressed is that people actively engaged with the epistemological and social dimensions of different bodies of knowledge. As I have argued, Pentecostal truth was about gaining a hold over elusive forces, about asserting one's own agency. The notion that divine intervention can be invoked through prayer was empowering in and of itself. It gave people the motivation to try to overcome their addictions, the confidence to search for a job. It provided direction in a context of post-Soviet chaos, in a situation of ideological excess. This logic also holds true for the ascent of Pentecostal Christianity in Kyrgyzstan more generally. It was asserting its own presence by claiming to make an impact on society, by seeking challenges. The Church of Jesus Christ was a forward-pushing movement, and could survive only by staying on the offensive. Numerous people fell by the wayside, but that was only to be expected because not everyone is chosen to be saved. In a sense, failure was part of the struggle between good and evil in this world, and it was through this struggle that a fragile conviction could be maintained.

6

The Tenacity of Spiritual Healing and Seeing

My friend Nurgul and I were seated on *tyshyks* (Kyrgyz, cotton mats) that were arranged along three walls of a small room, while Dinara prepared the low table in the middle for the séance. Nurgul had visited Dinara on earlier occasions, most recently when needing advice about the health problems of her cow, and she considered Dinara to be one of the stronger spiritual practitioners in Kokjangak. Dinara was a middle-aged woman of mixed Tatar and Russian descent and a self-declared *ekstra-sens* (someone with extrasensory perception). She was not surprised that a foreigner had come to consult her, because, she told us, many of her clients traveled from afar. Dinara took out prayer beads (*mishbaba*) and several stones, which she then moved slowly across the low table in circles and ellipses.

While performing her trade, Dinara described several of my personal characteristics quite accurately. However, when she declared that I was jobless and wanted to have my confirmation for this, I had no option but to object. A short but tense silence filled the room. Dinara turned toward

Nurgul, pointed to the stones, and said, "Here it clearly says that he does not have a job!" Luckily Nurgul offered her own insights, saying, "Well, you know, he doesn't get paid, he is like a volunteer; what he is doing is more like a hobby."[1] Dinara seemed relieved and replied, still somewhat grudgingly, "That must be it, because I clearly see that he doesn't have a *real* job."

Approximately half an hour later we left the house. Nurgul reflected on why Dinara might have been wrong.[2] She pondered that perhaps because I was a foreigner Dinara had been unable to connect with my psyche in the way she connected with other clients. "Anyway," she added, "you can never be certain. A year ago she healed my mother's eye disease, but perhaps she has lost her powers since." This was not the end of speculations. A week later Nurgul reported that she had run into Dinara, who had told Nurgul that she had sensed that I had "powers," and suspected that I had used those to obstruct her supernatural gifts. She advised Nurgul to be careful around me.

Why did the misinterpretation matter so much to both Nurgul and Dinara? Much was at stake in detecting the truth about spiritual forces in Kokjangak because, I will argue, the position of spiritual practitioners was anything but secure, and belief in spiritual power was anything but self-evident and stable. Moreover, these uncertainties resonated with the unpredictability that characterizes the spiritual forces concerned.

The foundation of spiritual healing and seeing in Kokjangak was unstable for three basic reasons. First, Dinara's troubled response to the failed vision and her attempt to influence Nurgul's interpretation of it illustrate the insecure position of individual practitioners. They did not occupy a formal office, and hence their reputation was dependent on interactions with clients as well as on talk about them among (potential) clients. For this reason practitioners needed to be constantly attentive to the signals they gave and the information that circulated about them in the community. Uncertainty regarding the qualities of individual practitioners was of direct concern to clients, especially to those who made significant payments or depended on spiritual practitioners for medical treatment or for guidance about important decisions. This was all the more critical because, as was common knowledge, there were many charlatans among the healers, who were in it for the money but did not actually have any extrasensory powers. Through interaction with clients, spiritual practitioners achieved, failed to achieve, or lost their reputation among their clients and the population more generally. The result of this was a dance around the notions of authenticity, rationality, and mystery, in which mediums tried to project, and clients detect, truth. And yet complete certainty always remained out of reach.

Another source of spiritual practitioners' instability concerns the phenomenon of "shamanic ideas and practices" more generally. The very reason for asking Nurgul to accompany me to Dinara was that as an educated foreigner I would have raised too many suspicions if not properly introduced.[3] Even if these two women did not question the reality of spiritual powers, their efforts to explain the failure implicitly conjured the skepticism about such powers among many others, especially members of the "intelligentsia." Dismissive attitudes may have been particularly pronounced in mining towns such as Kokjangak where the Soviet discourses of modernity and rationality had previously found strong resonance. But these dismissive attitudes were not just a legacy of the Soviet past. Spiritual practices were also condemned by representatives of new Islamic and Christian movements who saw the practices respectively as ineffective superstition or as satanic in origin. We will review these challenges in more detail below; for now it suffices to say that the field of spiritual healing and seeing was undergoing significant changes itself.

Third, the actions of *jinns* (ghosts or spirits) and the effects of mediation were themselves unpredictable. Spiritual practitioners such as Dinara acknowledged that they did not fully understand or control these forces. As alluded to above, I personally could well have brought new forces to Kokjangak, thereby altering the spiritual field. Moreover, because much of the spiritual world escapes our direct senses, and because spirits are capricious beings that do not act rationally but can be consumed by feelings of revenge, envy, and love, assessments made by spiritual practitioners were by definition tentative. Practitioners were but modest individuals acting within an overwhelming and capricious spiritual world that did not have a centered logic. Ironically, this form of instability actually strengthened the claims of practitioners (by making them less vulnerable to falsification) and thereby somewhat stabilized the spiritual field as a whole.

When these observations are applied to this book's overarching theme of the power of ideas, it becomes apparent that with these forms of spiritual healing and seeing we have entered terrain whose dynamics differ significantly from those discussed in previous chapters. In contrast to organized forms of religion and nonreligion, the spiritual practices discussed in this chapter lacked these obvious forms of institutionalization. While this made spiritual practitioners easy targets for the critiques of atheist activists, pastors, and imams, it also meant that such critiques had only limited effect.

Equally important is to point out that the spiritual practitioners were no missionaries or activists attempting to convince others of an absolute truth. Nor should their clients be seen as strong believers who reached (temporary) collective conviction. Rather, everyone involved moved within a space characterized by multilayered uncertainty: practitioners gained and lost status, clients became more and less convinced, specific ideas were easily taken up and discarded. Instead of assuming that belief in spirits simply exists, the relation between subjects and ideas is a dynamic one, and interdependent with the actions of multiple actors. Focusing on these actions and interactions will not provide direct access to people's "belief," but it will show how "believability" is produced. In this chapter, therefore, I analyze the discourses and actions of spiritual healers, their clientele, and other actors, to show how the believability of spiritual healers and clairvoyants is socially mediated and experientially constituted.[4]

Proliferation of Spiritual Practices

A wide range of terms was used to describe spiritual practitioners and their practices, often without much consistency. This terminological opacity was itself reflective of the uncertainty of the times and the range of influences that informed the practices. In offhand references, the most common general term for "spiritual practitioner" was *bakshi*. This term *bakshi* has its roots in the Chinese Empire where it referred to scribes, wizards, and Buddhist priests. From there it traveled first north to Siberia where it became a term for shaman, and then to Central Asia where it came to denote an Islamized shaman (Zarcone 2013, xxv). The Central Asian *bakshis*, in contrast to Siberian shamans, do not perform intercession on behalf of the community, nor do they travel to the other world. Instead they negotiate or fight with the spirits that roam in this world (Garrone 2013, 18, 27; Zarcone 2013, xxv). When I asked ordinary people in Kokjangak about the term, they would explain that *bakshis* are part of *kyrgyzchylyk* (the Kyrgyz way), that they lean toward shamanism, and that their practices involve fire and dark magic.

Interestingly, the healers and seers who were involved in such practices tended to shy away from the term *bakshi*. One reason for their reluctance was similar to what Johan Rasanayagam (2006, 383) observed in nearby Andijan (across the border in Uzbekistan), where the negative connotations of the term from a reformist Islamic point of view formed an important reason for avoiding the term. But often reluctance to use the term was for the opposite reason, namely that the *bakshi* was an awe-inspiring figure.[5] From this perspective, referring to oneself as *bakshi* would be presumptuous, implying that a practitioner considered his or her powers to match those of the great *bakshis* of the past.

The labels that practitioners used more readily included *moldo, tavyp, emchi, közü-achyk*, and *ekstra-sens*. In part this formed a spectrum ranging from practitioners who fully identified with Islam to those who employed unconventional sources of spirituality, such as science fiction images. The term *moldo* is also a general term for "mullah," or person knowledgeable about Islam, but used in this context it referred to a healer who treats patients by reciting the Koran, a process by which relevant passages of the holy text make a connection with the patient's body and thereby cleanse it of evil. The terms *tavyp* and *emchi* both mean "healer": *tavyp* stems from the Arabic *tabib*, or doctor, while *emchi* stems from the Kyrgyz *em*, to cure.[6] Their healing practices sometimes involved recitations of the Koran, but more often involved blowing, spitting, and whipping to cast out evil spirits. *Közü-achyk* literally means "with opened eyes" and has its Russian variant in *gadalka* (fortune-teller), though *közü-achyks* often did more than forecast the future. They also used their visionary capabilities to diagnose the causes of specific problems (including health-related ones), and combined this with prayers or other healing acts that "opened the way" for their clients. *Ekstra-sens* refers literally to the extrasensory perception of the practitioners involved, and was used by both Russian and Kyrgyz practitioners.

The various terms were used to evoke different traditions. Thus, *emchi* and *tavyp* connoted Islamic tradition, *közü-achyk* and *bakshi* evoked a sense of Kyrgyzness, and *ekstra-sens* and *gadalka* were associated with Russians. However, many practitioners used more than one term to describe themselves, which illustrates that the terms did not indicate fixed professional traditions but rather overlapping and changing fields of spiritual practice.[7]

My initial interest in practices of spiritual healing and seeing derived from the negative attention they received from Christian pastors and Islamic leaders, just as previously these activities had been condemned by Soviet atheist modernists. Imam Talant (see also chapter 3) talked dismissively about the local *bakshis*. In his view these *bakshis* were to be considered swindlers (*aferisty*) who had placed themselves outside of Islam by going against the Koran. The problem, from his perspective, was that during Soviet times many people had failed to differentiate between "what the mullah says and what the *bakshi* says." He attributed this to their lack of knowledge, a result of Soviet repression, because of which "they think that it is all Islam." It was one of the factors that had motivated the imam to start teaching *yiman* (Kyrgyz, belief, also connotes "morality") classes in the schools. Equally negative, but from a different perspective, was Pastor Kadyrjan's view (see chapter 5) on spiritual activities. He saw Kokjangak as a place replete with dark occult forces, which to him indicated that the town was a satanic stronghold. His aim was to defeat Satan in his home territory, something that would constitute a major blow to his might, and thereby initiate a domino effect in the region.

Whether or not these religious leaders would ever succeed in their struggles against what they denounced as "occultism" or "shamanism," the lamented practices were definitely thriving in the 1990s and early 2000s. As others have noted, this was a period in which there was a " 'new wave' of bakshi activity" throughout Central Asia (Vuillemenot 2013, 60; Somfai Kara 2013, 55). Kokjangak had at least twenty spiritual practitioners who regularly received clients. Of the eight healers I got to know, only one had been active during Soviet times; all others had taken up this trade in the 1990s. As one male acquaintance told me: "During the Soviet period there were far fewer [practitioners] than now. We were hardly aware of them, but perhaps in the villages [people] knew about them." Moreover, he added, "Back then they did it secretly, not like now."

The theme of post-Soviet proliferation often surfaced in conversations with residents of Kokjangak. Right after the collapse of the Soviet Union interest in spiritual healing and seeing had surged. One middle-aged woman voiced the general idea as follows: "These *bakshis* sprang up like mushrooms after the Union fell. There was so much talk about them at the time. We were constantly hearing, 'Here they heal, there they heal.'" In the early 1990s there had been several occasions when bus trips were organized to cities in Uzbekistan's part of the Fergana Valley to enable inhabitants to attend the healing sessions of famous spiritual healers. And when traveling visionaries came to Kokjangak, many residents took the chance to speak with their ancestral spirits.

The way people spoke about these events suggested that at the time they were approached as the next "new" thing. But ten years later, these same ideas and practices were often met with cynicism; the power of healers and clairvoyants was definitely not accepted by all. This was particularly the case among my "not religious" acquaintances who tended to describe all spiritual healers as charlatans. As one of them mused during a conversation:

[In the early 1990s] the number of clairvoyants [*ekstra-sens*] and fortune-tellers [*gadalki*] was rising strongly because it was the transition period [*perekhodnyi* period]. For most people this was a very difficult time. They got sick and started to speak with spirits. If you look here in town, it was mostly poor people [who started to consult spiritual healers], the reason being that life was difficult and their psyches couldn't handle it. Second, it was a way to earn money.

However, even those who were adamant that it was all deception insisted that it had been different in the past. Several skeptics recollected that in their youth (in the 1950s or 1960s) they had witnessed the performances of *bakshis* who "had *real* power."[8] For example, my acquaintance Nurbek remembered that in his childhood (in the 1960s) he had seen the last *real* female *bakshi* (or *bübü*) who was active in the region. This woman lived in a nearby village and had been called on to cure a baby who had previously been taken to the doctors, but in vain. Nurbek: "We gave money and a chicken. She started to walk in circles, first slowly, then gaining speed. As if in ecstasy she jumped up and down meanwhile hitting everyone really hard [with a whip (*kamchy*)] . . . reciting certain phrases while she was jumping and beating." Nurbek ascribed real powers to this *bakshi*, but added that nowadays no one possessed similar abilities. In short, there appeared to be a shared acknowledgment of the possibility of extrasensory powers, though people disagreed on whether contemporary healers and seers could mobilize them.

The correlation between socioeconomic disruption and spiritual activity was also reflected by the fact that many practitioners lived in the center of town, that is, in the part that had transformed most abruptly into an industrial wasteland. The rise of spiritual activities thus mirrored the inversion of social space. While in Soviet times the greatest density of spiritual practitioners had been in "backward" rural settings, now they resided primarily in the "chaotic" center of town. This is similar to Humphrey's argument that shamans were particularly important in the chaotic and impersonal post-Soviet urban environment, valued for their ability to reintegrate individuals in space and time (1999, 5).

Encounters between Healers and Clients

With the "real *bakshis*" perhaps no longer around, yet with the possibility of spiritual power looming large, it would be problematic to speak about belief as if it were a stable quality. Once again we are confronted with questions about truth and falsity. Such questions are discomforting for anthropologists because they easily result in either reductionist (positivistic) logic or in the collapse of critical distance. Yet the truth question needs to be engaged precisely because it was so relevant on the ground. It was well known that some self-proclaimed healers were in fact charlatans and imposters, and thus the claims of individual practitioners had to be scrutinized for possible fraud. Moreover, the existence of spirits and the possibility of their mediation were *not* taken for granted by many inhabitants, adding an additional layer of uncertainty to any truth quest. However, and somewhat counterintuitively, it was precisely this "doubtful" engagement with the possibility of truth that gave people's engagement with the world of spirits momentum.[9]

In looking at how truth is produced in spiritual healing and seeing, my approach was to accompany several acquaintances on their visits to spiritual healers. The advantage of this approach was that I could follow the process of motivation and deliberation, and document how authenticity and authority (or lack thereof) were created in interaction—both between client and practitioner and among clients. This approach offers only a partial view into the dynamics of belief, but it does generate important insight into how the conditions of belief—that is, believability—comes into being and disappears out of sight.

A revealing encounter was between Chinara and Marzia. Chinara, a thirty-eight-year-old Kyrgyz woman, worked for a local NGO in Kokjangak and held a degree from the University of Osh. She told me that as an educated woman she was skeptical about spiritual healing, especially because there were so many charlatans (*aferisty*). Nevertheless, she would occasionally visit a *bakshi*, which she justified by explaining that "still, they have a special kind of energy with which they can relieve you of stress." Chinara had known Marzia for a long time because the latter was a member of a credit and savings group she monitored as part of her job. In the past Marzia had offered to treat Chinara's headaches, and this occasion seemed a proper moment to accept the invitation. Before we arrived at Marzia's house Chinara told me some bits of information about Marzia's life that she considered particularly important: Marzia had been married three times and was raising two orphans in her home. To Chinara these two feats already indicated that Marzia was a special woman:[10]

> Women who become *bübü* or *bakshi* usually have some signs [Russian, *priznaki*]. Because they cannot find their place in life, they are not always able to find a reliable spouse, so they often end up being divorced. And with Marzia too, this is her third husband. . . . That is a general problem for all [spiritually gifted people], since there is an extra pressure on their psyche.

After we entered Marzia's house and were served tea, Marzia told me that her grandfather had been an important *tavyp* (healer) and that she had received powers through him. She had not known about these powers until, one day, she had become very ill. Friends suggested that she should see a *moldo*, but she didn't see the point and went to the hospital instead. She became paralyzed and could not leave her bed for a year, until a *moldo* started treating her. This *moldo*, for his part, insisted that Marzia should accept the powers he had detected in her, because otherwise she would become paralyzed again.[11]

We were seated in the living room. In the middle was a *shyrdak* (felt carpet) with a white cloth on top. Displayed on the white cloth were a whip and a bead chain. At the edge stood several cups with salt, others with tea leaves, and a few plastic bottles filled with water, which had been left there by some clients to absorb good powers.[12] The women sat down on the white cloth. Marzia instructed Chinara to relax and started her treatment. Marzia rhythmically hit Chinara with a whip, once in a while burping to release the bad energy she extracted from Chinara. She murmured words that were only occasionally audible enough to understand: "I am not God, I am not a prophet, but let the powers that I have support me in my actions," and "Let my actions serve the purpose to heal."[13] After the session or séance (*seans*) was finished, Marzia took her bead chain to read Chinara's state of being. I present here Chinara's rendering of what she had been told:

> It turns out that I am being protected by [a spirit in the guise of] a young man. He is jealous, and because of that my relationships with men fail to work out, that is why they won't stay around. I first have to ask [this young man] permission to marry; only then will it be possible for me to find someone, to fall in love, and to marry. And really, it is always with me like that. First, something happens, and then it won't work out. Maybe it is really true.
>
> [As I told you before] my grandmother from father's side . . . is related to water spirits, and now [Marzia] tells me that I have water spirits. She told me that I need to have this treatment more often; otherwise I will pass [the problems] on to my children. She also told me: "In the near future you will get a paper that will make you happy, and will increase your money." . . . That I have these people-spirits and that I need to prevent it from being passed on to my children—those are the things that I hear constantly. But what really surprised me was what she said about water spirits.

When we got back to Chinara's office, her assistant told her that the provincial government (Kyrgyz, *akimiat*) had called—they had received a fax from Bishkek saying that President Akaev was about to visit the province and that Chinara was expected to give a talk about her organization's work. Naturally, Chinara saw this as a confirmation of the forecasting powers of Marzia.[14] But more than this, it was the link that Marzia had made between her and her grandmother that she saw as significant. Although on an earlier occasion Chinara had dismissed the stories of her grandmother as fairy tales, through this encounter and Marzia's explanations these stories appeared to gain in significance.

My friend Nurgul has already been mentioned at the beginning of this chapter. A Kazakh woman of twenty-four, she had moved back in with her parents the year before when her short-lived marriage unraveled because of the increasingly abusive behavior of the man who was still officially her husband. The parental home was a modest house on the edge of the town center, surrounded by a small apple orchard. This was where she took care of her daughter while doing the housework, which was quite a burden because her mother had moved back to her natal village in Kazakhstan, at least for the time being. She often consulted clairvoyants and told me that she, her sister, and her daughter had all been healed by a Catholic *ekstra-sens* of Polish background (who did not agree to meet me). Together we decided to visit Gulnara, about whose powers Nurgul had heard positive stories, although she had never visited Gulnara before.

Gulnara's house showed few visual signs indicating she was a spiritual healer—there were, for example, no items left by clients or religiously inspired pictures. When I asked Gulnara what she would call herself, she pondered the question for a second and then replied that she was an *ekstra-sens*, because she not only saw things but also healed, took away spells, and "opened" people's future. She said that even when she was a schoolgirl, she had already cured people: "They would come with a little child. I simply washed [these little children], and within three days, they would be better." At the time she didn't recognize her gift, and for the rest of her youth and early adulthood she did not actively engage in spiritual practices.

When she turned fifty, however, she experienced a change in her physique. For days on end she felt as if she was engulfed by waves, during which she started to see people no one else could see. She found out that these people—she described them as humans—were from outer space and wanted to teach her how to perform medical treatments. Gulnara had to remain indoors for forty days, during which she was taught the alien physicians' skills. Among the skills she had thus acquired she counted giving injections from her fingertips as well as more complex treatments such as transfusing blood and other substances in order to replace polluted body liquids. While treating her patients she often consulted these alien physicians and sometimes left it to them to perform the surgery, especially when the risks of complications were high.

Nurgul volunteered to be examined. She had to lie down on the carpet (*shyrdak*) in the middle of the room and close her eyes. Gulnara moved her hands up and down Nurgul's body, following her curves, sometimes halting and pressing her hands onto the skin to examine more closely. The examination lasted about fifteen minutes. Nurgul was declared healthy, apart from a backache and an excessive level of stress. Gulnara explained that although during the examination she had already taken away some of the accumulated stress, Nurgul would have to come back for a series of treatments if she wanted to get rid of it completely.

After we left the house, Nurgul mentioned that she had felt shivers of coldness when Gulnara touched her. She felt this energy also in the room, and these experiences convinced her that Gulnara had real powers and was not a charlatan. I asked her what she thought about the physicians from the other planet. She said:

> For me this is nothing new. I have discussed these things often with my neighbor [who also was an *ekstra-sens*]. You know, Americans have a lot of movies, fantasy movies, and these are about energy, about mutants, phantoms. Someone must put it in the heads of the movie directors, right? It is not simply that they make it up. For example, no matter how much fantasy you have, you won't come up with a movie like *The Matrix*.

The Believability of Spiritual Practices

Both cases illustrate how the believability of spiritual healers and seers is mediated by the experiences, memories, hopes, and fears of their clients. Being reminded of what Grandmother once said, receiving a sign of impending prosperity, being confronted with the possibility of future loneliness—these all provided strong incentives for being favorably disposed to the messages of the practitioners. The practitioners made personal experiences such as divorce or poverty understandable by embedding them in larger fields of power, even if the features of the forces involved could not be fully understood. Further reflections on these issues provide insight into why people sought advice or treatment, and how the efficacy of particular healing and seeing practices was dialogically produced.

Reasons for Seeking Treatment

There were many reasons why residents sought the services of spiritual healers and clairvoyants. They were rooted in the uncertainties of existence, based on an awareness or at least an inkling that spirits actively influence daily life, and on the possibility that these spirits could be manipulated for good and bad.

Unsurprisingly, health problems were the most common reason for seeing a clairvoyant or spiritual healer. In some cases the client had received biomedical treatment at the hospital without obtaining the desired effect and visited a spiritual healer as a last resort. Financial considerations clearly played a role. As one woman said: "When I go to the hospital, they just ask for money—money, money, money. You need to pay for everything: for registration, for seeing the doctor, for treatment."[15] Deterioration of health services was also mentioned. One middle-aged man told me: "You know, during the Soviet period we had excellent health care. But they sold all the equipment, so what kind of treatment do you expect?" The message, apparently, was that spiritual healing provided better value for money (which is not to say that choosing one or another form of treatment was based on explicit calculations).

Aside from the monetary aspect, an important consideration in deciding which treatment to seek was the cause of a health problem. Whenever the problem was obviously caused by an accident or was a known medical condition, most people would first go to the hospital or medical point. Other problems, such as rashes, backaches, headaches, impotency, and infertility, were thought to be more effectively treated by spiritual healers. However, it was often difficult to determine the cause of a health problem. In fact, numerous physical problems—but also social ones such as joblessness, bad luck in business, and so on—could have been caused by someone having cast a spell on you, or by spirits who had latched on to you, as was the case with Chinara.

A Russian healer explained to me how to find out if a spell has been cast on you as follows: "When you have a feeling that things do not work out as they should, but you don't understand the reason—then it is *koldovstvo* [sorcery]." She added that you can detect it inside yourself as something that feels unsettled and out of place. In some instances people were confronted with concrete evidence of the casting of such a spell, as in the case of a young woman whose mother-in-law cursed her in public after she had decided to divorce her husband. Other examples included the following: a woman explained that she knew a spell had been cast on her when she found dry sand in front of her door; another told me she had found thin black threads tied into knots under her desk at work. This type of dry sand and the black knots were known to have been prepared by *bakshis* or other practitioners who engaged in dark magic (*chernoe koldovstvo*). Though such literal proofs of *koldovstvo* were not uncommon, the suggestion that magic was involved often came from a third person (a friend or relative) who had witnessed changes in the behavior, appearance, or mood of the victim. In a way, then, the significance of spiritual healing was produced by social communication on the nature and causes of specific problems. A general awareness of the potential of spiritual powers was constantly being regenerated, and even skeptics were not immune to the ideas.

This backdrop is important for understanding the popularity of spiritual healing in general, but it does not explain the values that people attached to the concrete treatments of individual healers. In fact, everyone knew there were some imposters, and hence there was no certainty concerning the actual powers of individual healers. This brings us to the question of how healers tried to establish their authority.

Appeals to Authority

In her discussion of spiritual healing in contemporary Russia, Lindquist (2001) refers to Weber's typology of the three main sources of authority—rational-legal, traditional, and charismatic—and their adaptation by Carol MacCormack to the medical field, in order to arrive at a typology that makes sense for understanding the legitimizing strategies of spiritual healers in Moscow. These are (1) rational-legal, based on diplomas, documents, and formal education; (2) traditional, based on ties to the past and the invocation of tradition; and (3) alterity, or otherness, in which healers "draw on their own versions of globality" and are seen as mediators between the local and the global.

Appeals to rational-legal or bureaucratic authority were of minor consequence in Kokjangak. Whereas Lindquist (2001) has shown how in Moscow newspaper advertisements were used to foster an image of efficiency—by showing healers in a suit and tie or by mentioning degrees from official medical schools—such images would not have counted for much in Kokjangak. In fact, the town once received a visit from two men who called themselves representatives of a medical school in Bishkek and claimed they were designated to register the spiritual healers, offering them official certificates in exchange for money. Although one of the local healers told me that she had been impressed by the appearance of these men, neither she nor anyone else had bothered to obtain the "official certificates." It seemed that the dilapidated condition of official institutions in the region—among which were educational and medical structures—led to a situation in which spiritual healers distanced themselves from official biomedical medicine and certainly did not want to pay money for certificates.

Appeals to *traditional* authority did play an important role in the way healers and clairvoyants presented themselves. This was evident from Marzia's mention that her grandfather had been an important healer, invoking the term *tavyp* that signified an acknowledged position within the Islamic community. In other instances this invocation of tradition was visible in the display of posters of Mecca or, in the case of a Russian healer, icons, paintings of Jesus, and postcards showing the Virgin Mary. The connection with "tradition" also surfaced when Chinara evaluated the spiritual powers of Marzia. The way people described Marzia reminded her of the stories told by her grandmother in her youth, which, although her educational background urged her to regard them as fantasy, continued to be more than just "fairy tales." Likewise, many people skeptical of contemporary spiritual healers made a differentiation between the powerful *bakshis* of the past and the charlatans of today. Claims of genealogical links to such recognized healers of the past and displays of traditional healing elements such as knucklebones, horse whips, or blessed water (see also Penkala-Gawęcka 2013, 41) were common, even if not always successful, ways of addressing such skepticisms.

In order to claim special powers for dealing with spirits, healers also appealed to registers of otherness, or *alterity*. Almost all spiritual healers presented their biography as exceptional, thereby describing themselves as

partial outsiders to the local community. The idea here was that only people who were born with special gifts, and had gone through extraordinary
episodes of suffering, were able to engage effectively with the spirits, and to
mediate between different worlds. These claims to alterity were often cast
within the framework of tradition. Thus, Marzia's story of having become
paralyzed, of initially resisting her spiritual gifts, and finally accepting
them together with the consequence of remaining unmarried, consisted
of narrative elements that circulate widely among healers.[16] Apart from
making use of traditional elements, the displays of alterity could also make
use of other registers. Gulnara's stories were a case in point. Although her
recounting of illness was a familiar trope, most of the elements in her presentation were novel ones, including spaceships, UFOs, and alien doctors.
To some of my acquaintances this proved she was a nutter, but to Nurgul
and presumably most of Gulnara's clients it demonstrated that she was a
powerful mediator between different worlds.

Ascribing and Contesting Believability

The described practices and self-portrayals illustrated how healers tapped
into several registers of authority and incorporated elements from contemporary consumer culture. But while these self-portrayals were certainly
commented on when clients assessed the worth of various healers, they
were not decisive in such assessments. Although both Chinara and Nurgul included images of tradition and otherness in their evaluation of the
healers' spiritual powers, this is not to say that they were always convinced
by the appeals to those registers of authority. The risk of forgery or deception was simply too high. Moreover, because Kokjangak was a small town
where word-of-mouth information about individuals spread quickly, the
self-presentations of healers were perhaps less important than the way they
were talked about among friends, neighbors, and colleagues. Ultimately,
the practitioners' believability depended on how their effectiveness in forecasting and healing was communicated by members of the community.

The practitioners themselves tried to demonstrate their efficacy by
telling stories of the number of people they had healed, by stressing the
severity of diseases, and by mentioning that they attracted clientele from
faraway places. However, they were well aware that their forecasts and
treatments would not always live up to expectations. When confronted

with such cases they pointed out various reasons for failure. The most common explanation was that the client had not followed instructions properly. Another was that a new spell had been cast on the client, demanding further and more intensive treatment. Interestingly enough, such spells could also affect the practitioner's powers (as in the example at the beginning of this chapter), so that their visionary and healing capacities were temporarily blocked by the spell of another healer or clairvoyant. Nurgul told me once how amazed she was that the healers "constantly try to obstruct each other's powers." She recalled a story of her *ekstra-sens* neighbor who complained that other healers had extracted her energy and that after one particular encounter she had been sick for two days. Nurgul laughed when telling me this story and said that she was happy not to be a healer herself.

Even among those who consult healers and seers there was a constant pondering over whether to believe the forecasting and healing powers of the practitioners. For instance, Asia, a woman in her late thirties, told me that although some people had real powers, there was a lot of forgery involved. She explained:

> About a year ago I went with a friend to this healer [Marzia]. She said: "It turns out that your road is blocked, they obstructed your road. That is why you won't marry." And then she said: "I will open your road. You should bring a new lock, a chicken, three meters of good cloth, and three bars of soap—actually it should be seven but I will ask only three." When we were outside my friend said that she wouldn't go to her again because [Marzia] was obviously trying to pull her leg. We went to another one [for a second opinion] and were told: "Don't worry. Although there was *koldovtsvo*, it is already leaving you."

In this case, the vision provided by the first clairvoyant (Marzia) was "falsified" by alleging greediness, which to Asia and her friend indicated that she was concerned only with her own material needs. Asia later suggested that Marzia had probably invented the story of the friend's obstructed road so that she could offer expensive treatment. Likewise, Nurgul, who figured earlier in this chapter, told me that she often tested the analyses of particular clairvoyants. Whenever there was a discrepancy she would basically choose the most plausible one. Since such stories about healing effectiveness were communicated among friends and neighbors, a very loose and shifting differentiation emerged in the powers attributed to individual healers.

Animating the Urban Wasteland

One of Nurgul's neighbors had been trying to sell her house for over half a year. She needed to sell badly because the whole family was moving to the north, so she had made a large sign saying "for sale." The house was in a good location, at the edge of the center, in reasonable condition, with a sizable orchard and a small barn. In her view, it was logical to expect an interested party to come forward soon. But not a single person had made inquiries. Through consultation with a *közü-achyk* she discovered that someone had been blocking the path to her house, diverting potential buyers from even noticing the "for sale" sign. She was hoping that the *közü-achyk*'s efforts to remove the blockage were strong enough, and that the person who had blocked the road would not create new obstacles.

The proliferation of spiritual activity was rooted in disruption, linked to socioeconomic destabilizations and the effects these had on people's everyday life. Healers did more than heal and clairvoyants offered more than glimpses of what the future might hold. They also made the postindustrial urban environment meaningful or comprehensible, explaining why one might fail to sell a house, for instance. The cityscape was not just background for the spiritual practices; the two were closely interwoven. As Caroline Humphrey has argued in her paper "Shamans in the City," the practitioners "themselves 'actualize space' . . . and thereby create new contexts of the city" (2002, 203–4). By displaying their visions, the clairvoyants provided livable explanations for the hardship that people in Kokjangak experienced. Whereas an outsider might ascribe these difficulties simply to the asymmetries and destabilizing effects of the new economy, the clairvoyants managed to translate such abstract forces to more immediate causes that explained individual stories of success and failure.

Thus, the fact that someone did not manage to sell her house was attributed to the spiritual obstruction of the road leading to that house, while other visions explained why a suitable marriage partner was unavailable (in a place where labor migration had produced a deficit of men). Although these visions provided meaning and hope to individuals who were suffering, the clairvoyants' visions for the city as a whole were often far

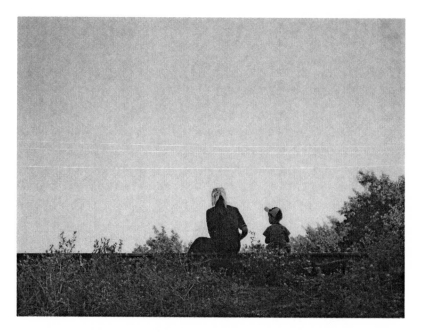

Mother and son, August 2009

from rosy. Two of the clairvoyants with whom I was acquainted took their visions to a more prophetic level. For them, observations of UFOs, pervasive corruption, and the general decline of Kokjangak signaled that the end of times was nigh.

Tenacity

In the beginning of this chapter I proposed to differentiate between three levels of instability, each of which affect the ideas and practices related to spiritual healing and seeing in Kokjangak. One level of instability concerns suspicion of the claims of individual *bakshis* and the possibility of fraud, which resulted in a dance around ideas of truth and authenticity. Another level concerned the capricious behavior of spirits, the complex relationships among spirits and among *bakshis*, making the relationship between the world of the spirits and the human world an unpredictable one. Ironically, the unpredictability and complexity somewhat stabilized the position of the practitioners, because failures of vision or cure could have been caused as much by the inabilities of the practitioners as by the unpredictability of the world of spirits. As we saw, the latter possibility was actively pursued by some of the practitioners as well as some of the clients. This resulted in a flexible space in which there was no complete certainty about any position—a space of ambiguity in which ideas of self and society emerged and were actively discussed (see also Louw 2010).

The question that was left somewhat hanging in the air was how these two levels of instability intersect with the second level of instability, related to external challenges to spiritual practices. During Soviet times the practices of clairvoyants, shamans, and other spiritual practitioners had been denounced as backward superstition. Obviously not everyone had bought into Soviet modernist logic, and the *bakshi* remained a known figure, part of "Kyrgyz tradition" (*kyrgyzchylyk*). But in urban contexts their position had become marginal and unimportant, as the recollections of inhabitants testified. Secularization was not just a myth: the image of modernity that had been so consciously cultivated in Soviet Kokjangak fostered skepticism about spiritual practitioners. Moreover, the Soviet welfare system made life trajectories more predictable and secure, which, together with the availability of free biomedical health services, meant there was less demand for the consultations and treatments of spiritual practitioners. The Soviet experiment had marginalized and destabilized spiritual practices but did not eradicate them.

The popularity of healers and clairvoyants partly stemmed from the severe socioeconomic crisis and the resulting uncertainties for individuals. Furthermore, their authority was enhanced by the loss of credibility that secular ideologies faced after the collapse of socialism. Certainly, "not religious" and self-proclaimed "modern" inhabitants continued to denounce what they saw as superstitious practices. The physicians and head nurses at the hospital were most explicit in their criticism and in stressing detrimental health consequences of reliance on spiritual healers. But their credibility was limited because the hospital was in disarray and, realistically speaking, hardly offered better medical care than some of the spiritual healers. Moreover, the "secular" critiques of spiritual healers were often undermined by the ambivalence of the secularists themselves, who valued the "spiritual" images of Kyrgyz history and admitted that among the charlatans and impostors were those with real powers.

The more imminent challenges to the described ideas of spirituality came increasingly not from secular voices but from religious ones. This trend has been reported across Central Asia. Thus, David Somfai Kara writes about Kazakhstan and Kyrgyzstan that "in recent years fundamentalist Muslims have begun to put forward the idea that all these traditions should be excluded from religious practices, because they are not part of 'real' Islam" (2013, 53; see also Louw 2010). And speaking about Central Asia as a whole, Thierry Zarcone writes that "shamans are fiercely fought by orthodox Islam and especially by its radical wing, Wahhabism" (2013, xxvi). The situation was not different in Kokjangak, where the imam was one of the active agitators against what he described as "national customs." The imam presented his view in the mosque as well as in the classes on religious history and morality (Kyrgyz, *yiman sabaq*) that he taught at one of the schools. He knew that members of the older generation were often skeptical about his views, but he had success among a growing group of young men and women who were attracted to a purer and more pious form of Islam than what they had experienced at home.

And then there was the Pentecostal church headed by Pastor Kadyrjan, who had decided that "occultism" was the biggest obstacle to establishing a viable church in Kokjangak. The church did not dismiss local healing practices as ineffective superstition (as atheism did, and to some extent reformist Islam). Rather, "occult" practices were interpreted as being linked to Satan and thus part of a larger spiritual warfare in which Pentecostal Christians were fighting on the side of God. This also suggests that there were remarkable similarities between the worldview promoted by Pentecostals and indigenous notions about spirits, as well as between Christian faith healing (as discussed in chapter 5) and the healing practices described in this chapter. The rapid growth of Pentecostalism in the early 2000s can be partly ascribed to its affinities with existing notions about the world of spirits, and partly to its more centralized forms of communication. Why indeed did the converts of chapter 5 feel that through Jesus they were more likely to achieve their goals than through spiritual healers? One answer is that the Pentecostals were better organized and more effective in promoting their success stories than spiritual healers were. The church actively encouraged interpreting positive events as gifts of God and as examples demonstrating the effectiveness of prayer. Moreover, in church services and home-church meetings people were literally taught to interpret their experiences in terms of Pentecostal thought. The Pentecostal Church, just like reformist Islam, was able to rely on institutional structures in the communication of truths.[17] By contrast, the spiritual practitioners were on their own, and in fact actively undermined each other's claims to authority.

Both reformist Islam and Pentecostal Christianity were gaining influence, in part because they could rely on institutional structures in delivering their messages, and also because of their more rigid denunciations of corruption and immorality. Moreover, whereas for many spiritual healers the economic and social crises in Kokjangak signaled the end of times, the new Islamic and Pentecostal visions had a more hopeful message. In their view, the crisis resulted from old corruptions (spiritual and social) to which their religions claimed to provide effective answers.

However, the fact that spiritual practitioners could not and did not advance "grand and hopeful promises" may also indicate their strength. The status of such practitioners depended on individual claims to legitimacy, and on informal channels that alternately stressed or challenged their effectiveness. This unstable basis of authority was in part their strength because it provided room for the negotiation of meaning and allowed for a flexible hierarchy among clairvoyants and healers. The healers may not have had the institutional mechanisms to advance a master narrative, but neither were they the prisoners of such grand narratives. In a society where the narrative of socialism had vanished and the rhetoric of capitalism, modernity, and transition turned out to be hollow, new grand ideologies or doctrines seemed to be destined to lead to disillusionment as well. That is, the smaller stories, the contextualized messages that relate the present to the past, give meaning to locality, and root individuals in their world, may prove more believable than the grand narratives. And if not, then they can easily be adjusted.

CONCLUSION

Pulsation and the Dynamics of Conviction

pulsation noun | pul·sa·tion | \ ˌpəl-ˈsā-shən\ 1: rhythmical throbbing or
vibrating (as of an artery); *also*: a single beat or throb 2: a periodically
recurring alternate increase and decrease of a quantity (as pressure, volume,
or voltage)

The relationship between power and collective ideas is riddled with contradictions. The ideas that are most conspicuously present, that are most
aggressively pushed, are also the most likely to collapse under their own
weight. Seen from the opposite angle, ideas that form an integral part of
society tend to be taken for granted, and as such lack the ability to stir people's feelings, to motivate inspired action. Collective ideas can be motivational only when there is a tension—due to a discrepancy with reality or
caused by challenges to their integrity—which makes them worthy and in
need of propagation or defense. It is due to this dynamic that conviction
thrives in contexts of instability. In other words, the potency of ideology is
rooted in its fragility.

In this book we have explored the relationship between sociopolitical
instability and conviction through an examination of how secular and religious collective ideas fared in conditions of existential uncertainty, paying
attention to the hopes they instilled and the actions they inspired among

residents of a destitute former mining town, as well as to the suspicions, skepticisms, and disillusions these same ideas evoked. I have described the precarious attempts of "secularists" to position themselves between fading Soviet atheism and assertions of new forms of religiosity; the successes and failures in the activities of Tablighi Muslims as they moved into "uncharted" territory, and of a Pentecostal church on the religious frontier; and how spiritual practitioners who were sometimes labeled "shamans" operated in unpredictable spiritual fields. With the ethnographic engagements behind us it will be worthwhile to provide further reflections on the dynamics of conviction, to outline a conceptual framework that is capable of illuminating how collective ideas gain and lose force.

The term "pulsation" is such a productive metaphor for talking about conviction because it highlights that impermanence and fluctuation are key characteristics of ideational power. As in the above definition from *Merriam-Webster's*, it is possible to distinguish between at least three aspects. Pulsation begins with the "single beat or throb," that is, with the impulse that sets things in motion. In the realm of ideas this translates to a reaching out, a "voicing of hope" that is simultaneously a yearning for and a conceptualization of a utopian horizon. Second, the impulse needs to gain traction (or find pressure points to push against) if it is to produce an increase of "pressure or voltage." This tends to happen when ideas are seen as relevant and important, which means that they should be neither completely taken for granted nor completely outrageous. Finally, even if one beat released in the right environment may produce a ripple, for collective ideas to be characterized by a "rhythmical throbbing or vibrating" the impulses or beats need to arrive in appropriate intervals or reverberate within a group of people.

Together these three aspects make up the process by which meaningful ideas attain affective and effervescent qualities, that is, by which ideas are endowed with a sense of not only truth, but also of imminence, importance, and justice. But while these dynamics should be seen as working in an ensemble, it should also be noted that they are never in complete harmony. The production of conviction is a delicate undertaking with distinctive temporal characteristics and limits. At each of the points—the voicing, the responding, the reverberating—things can and do go wrong.

Voicing Hope on the Frontier

> The frontier was not the end ("tail") but rather the beginning ("forehead") . . .
> it was the spearhead of light and knowledge expanding into the realm of
> darkness and the unknown . . . pioneer settlements of a forward moving
> culture bent on occupying the whole area.
>
> Ladis K. D. Kristof (1959, 270)

Kristof's historical definition of the frontier powerfully conveys the perspective of the settler, the pioneer, and the missionary as they look out over what to them appears as barren land, an expanse into which they can venture, and which they set out to appropriate by transforming it, a process through which they are themselves rejuvenated.[1]

This perspective reflects well how the various "ideologues" in this book talked about Kyrgyzstan and especially Kokjangak. International development specialists had seen Kyrgyzstan as a testing ground for neoliberal policies, with a population in need of being trained in the workings of the free market. An example that comes to my mind is from a day in Kokjangak back in 1999 when a visiting German UNDP colleague (who, like me, was in his twenties) was vigorously drawing business plans on a flip chart. He solicited ideas from his mostly female and visibly impoverished audience—to make and sell pastry, for example—then drew boxes and arrows to which he attached numbers and words, which together purported to demonstrate how the women's ideas could be turned into successful businesses. What his performance conveyed was the certainty that his approach was right and the conviction that it *would* bring prosperity to the poor.

This self-righteous attitude, which was based on a perceived contrast between the "spearhead of light" and the "realm of darkness," shone through even more strongly in my conversations with Pastor Kadyrjan. As the representative of a Pentecostal church that placed great emphasis on evangelism, he talked about Kokjangak as if it was the ultimate frontier, and elaborated in his sermons on the various evil spirits that still kept the town in their "ice cold" grip.[2] Conquering this town (in the sense of establishing a thriving congregation) would deliver a decisive blow to Satan, and thus not only save the lives of the converted but achieve an important victory for Jesus in the whole region.

On the frontier the differentials between perceived superiority and inferiority are simultaneously very pronounced *and* at risk of collapsing or inverting. The sense of superiority was reflected in the comportment of the "pioneers": the soft-spoken certainty of *amir* Nur Islam, the unreflective enthusiasm of my UNDP colleague, and the unwavering exclamations of Pastor Kadyrjan. This sense of superiority tends to grow, as it were, with each step deeper into the frontier as this reveals ever-larger contrasts with the pioneer's "civilization." And yet each step will make the pioneer more vulnerable, until he or she is either reduced to a voice in the desert or falls over to the other side. These dangers are recognized by the pioneers themselves, which makes reflecting on them all the more interesting.

The risk of failing to find an audience—of becoming a lone voice in the desert—is one that probably troubles most secular and religious missionaries as they set out on their missions. In light of this Simon Coleman has written that even when the missionary fails to convince others, they still "have an audience of at least one, given that the evangelical speaker is also perforce a listener, attending to a message that achieves an important part of its purpose merely by being powerfully and passionately projected out into the world" (2003, 24). Coleman's is a valuable observation, as it emphasizes the invigorating effect of doing missionary work, whether religious or political. But although an "audience of one" may be sufficient for some preachers, it is definitely not for all. During my last encounter with Gulbarchyn (the church leader who was sent by Pastor Kadyrjan to live and work in Kokjangak), we talked about the difficulty of living in a place whose residents were either hostile or indifferent to her presence, and about how her difficulties were confounded by the partial disintegration of the local congregation. To me she appeared despondent, and thus I was not surprised when the following year I was informed that Gulbarchyn had left Kokjangak to rejoin her family in Jalalabad city.

The other risk—of falling over to the other side—is one that perhaps speaks even more directly to the imagination. Just as anthropologists talk with a mix of intrigue and contempt about (former?) colleagues who ended up "going native," so do Christian and development missionaries about theirs. An evangelical example from Kyrgyzstan concerned Risbek, a US missionary who had fallen in love with Kyrgyz culture and become convinced that the Kyrgyz were one of the lost tribes of Israel. As proof for this idea he embarked on a lengthy study of the Manas epic, ultimately concluding that the epic was rooted in the Bible.[3] Risbek was controversial in evangelical circles because his ideas demonstrated to some that "contextualization" had turned into "syncretism," meaning that efforts to make the biblical message meaningful to a local population had ended up corrupting the message, which therefore was no longer biblical. A very different example is from my first days as a United Nations Volunteer (UNV), when I and several other new recruits were told the story of a colleague who had just been dismissed. This colleague had been working for several years in Kyrgyzstan's remote Batken area when, during an unannounced visit, UNDP officials found him spending his workday, accompanied by two young women, in a sauna illegally built with development money.

Even if they were not always successful, the movements discussed in this book had their own strategies for dealing with the dangers of the frontier. The Tablighi approach is particularly useful for illustrating adaptations to frontier conditions. Their *dawatchis*, or travelers, would never venture into the unknown alone and risk being swallowed up by the frontier. All their activities—traveling to new places, inviting people to the mosque, eating and sleeping—were carried out in the company of fellow travelers, which allowed the "voice of ideology" to resonate within the fellowship even when there was no external audience. When in 2010 I conversed with visiting *dawatchis* in the former mining town of Ak-Tiuz, they mentioned that two days into their *dawat* I was the first person to come to their makeshift mosque. To them this did not indicate that their mission was a failure, because even their mere presence would leave behind "spiritual footprints" and thereby prepare the ground for a future spiritual awakening.[4] Meanwhile, the *dawatchis'* own commitment to the true path was being strengthened by the confrontation with the horrors of life in a God-deserted place.

It is important to reemphasize that mining towns such as Kokjangak and Ak-Tiuz had not always been a "realm of darkness." In fact, until recently Kokjangak had been an outpost of Soviet modernity—its own "spearhead of light and knowledge" (to use Kristof's [1959] vocabulary once more). It used to be a well-off industrial town inhabited by people who considered themselves educated and cultured, some of whom would venture into the "backward" surrounding villages to battle the vestiges of religious traditions (chapter 3). The memories of this glorious past made the downfall into chaos all the more painful. But perhaps it is hardly surprising that the pioneers of Soviet modernity had become the post-Soviet targets of new civilizing missions. Painful as it was, the inversion is a reminder that frontiers are human constructs in which the dominant perspective gets to define "wildness," something that had radically altered with the collapse of the Soviet Union and its socialist and militantly secular ideology.[5] The town's modernist past also meant that Kokjangak inhabitants often saw themselves as more civilized than the missionaries who targeted them, with the result that while residents were on the one hand reaching out to new horizons, on the other they were often skeptical of new assertions of truth.

But I am getting ahead of myself. Let's first summarize some key points. Pulsation starts with a clear ideological "voice"—the impulse—which is a necessary precondition for having an effect. The frontier, which to the pioneer and ideologue contained the promise of expansion and transformation, triggered such clear voices. And yet the same frontier conditions challenged ideological clarity, with the voice of ideology running the risk of either cracking or being deafened out by its surroundings. In that sense the frontier is also a frontier between conviction and doubt.

Responding: Productive Tensions

> Friction is not just about slowing things down. Friction is required to keep global power in motion. . . . The effects of encounters across difference can be compromising or empowering.
>
> ANNA TSING (2005, 6)

Anna Tsing's statement about the need for friction to keep things moving applies not only to global power but has much broader applicability, as can be seen in the works of various thinkers. Not that they always use the word "friction" when talking about specific productive tensions. Slavoj Žižek speaks of the vital importance of "the obstacle," which, on the one hand, prevents the full deployment of productive forces but, on the other, is simultaneously the "condition of possibility" because a complete realization (of love, for example) would remove the mystery and thereby deflate interest (Žižek 2001, 18). Ernesto Laclau writes (2005, 85) about a broken space that separates the people from power, a gap or lack in the sociopolitical field that is a necessary condition for the formation of genuine populist movements. Arjun Appadurai speaks about the tension between the national ideal of homogeneity and the messy reality of a globalizing world, which produces an "anxiety of incompleteness" (2006). To return to the term "friction," Anna Tsing argues that notwithstanding popular talk of

a borderless world of flows, globalization "can only be charged and en-
acted in the sticky materiality of practical encounters" (2005, 1).[6] It would
not be difficult to expand this rather eclectic list, but the point is that "friction" is also a key dimension in the trajectory of ideas. Ideas only come
to matter—they "gain traction," as I formulated it above—when they are
not completely taken for granted, that is, when they are challenged, either
from within or from without.

Friction is ultimately about "encounters across difference" (Tsing 2005, 3),
which, applied to this book, concerns the tensions between people's dreams,
values, and ideas and the terrain onto which these are projected. Tsing
rightly argues that friction can be enabling as much as it can be compromis-
ing. Too much friction slows things down, while the lack of friction means
the loss of any grip.[7] In the pages below, I will draw on the ethnographic
evidence from this book to make tentative claims about the enabling and
disabling role of friction. Starting with tensions in the properties of the
advanced ideas themselves, attention will then move to discrepancies between these ideas and the realities of life as they are experienced.

Pascal Boyer's theory of "minimal counter-intuitiveness" posits that
concepts, images, and ideas are particularly appealing when they conform
to certain intuitive assumptions about a class of objects, while simultaneously violating some of those assumptions (1994, 3–5; see also Sperber
1985). In other words, for ideas to gain traction they should be neither
self-evident nor outlandish, but rather "thought provoking." There is no
need to enter the sterile debate as to whether or not "counter-intuitiveness"
reflects "non-cultural properties of the human mind-brain" as Boyer has
it (1994, 3) to recognize the relevance of the general principle for the study
of conviction. It suffices here to say that newly introduced ideas on the one
hand need to make sense, while on the other they need to "stand out." And
maintaining this balance is particularly important when the advanced ideas
cannot fall back on dominant social conventions or institutional structures.

The balance between uniqueness and familiarity has been a recurrent
theme in this book, coming across particularly vividly in the self-portrayals of
spiritual healers who, while presenting themselves as novel and exceptional,
simultaneously drew on established ideas of how spiritual healers are supposed to act. The example of Gulnara (chapter 6) is a good one to recall. Her
invocation of alien doctors and her use of invisible needles and other surgical
instruments were confounding to some of her patients, but she made these

digestible through her conventional story of becoming a "shaman," which explained how she had been inaugurated into the profession after a protracted illness and with the blessing of her spiritual teachers. The discussion of the liminal position of the Tablighi Jamaat pointed in the same direction. Here it was a trade-off between their unusual and foreign appearance and their connection with Soviet and Kyrgyz "nomadic" practices that produced a "minimal counter-intuitiveness" that proved attractive to many men.[8]

"Counterintuitiveness" refers to principles of classification and the dilemma of what to do with elements that do not fit classificatory schemes. It is important to emphasize that such schemes cannot be understood separately from the context in which they arise and are employed. As Mary Douglas pointed out quite a few decades ago, classificatory schemes are ultimately expressions of existing patterns of social relations, such that anomalies in those schemes tend to be understood as violations of the social order (1975, 249). While initially arguing that such violations are generally considered dangerous "dirt" that as "matter out of place" require removal (1966), in one of her later essays Douglas (1975) refined this idea, saying that the evaluation of anomalies in classificatory schemes correlates with the evaluation of the relations between a community and the surrounding world. When these external relations are negative, anomalies tend to be seen as problematic and dangerous. When relations with the outside are positive, anomalies tend to be imbued with positive or even sacred value. This then brings us to the question of how the tension between the ideal and the real can spark desire as well as anxiety.

Ghassan Hage (2003) has argued that the shrinking of the state—in his case the Australian state under neoliberal reform—undermines the capacity to generate and distribute hope among its population, a process in which citizens develop a "worrying attachment" to society that reveals itself in xenophobic sentiments and more generally a "paranoid nationalism" (3). The disarray of the state system in post-Soviet Kyrgyzstan similarly produced "worrying attachments" among citizens. This flared up with particular intensity in 2010, when the country's sovereignty was felt to be under threat, resulting in mass violence against the Uzbek minority. The positive revaluation of Soviet atheism made by "secularists" and their negative response to assertions of religiosity could similarly be interpreted as projecting fears stemming from their own marginalization onto "everything classified as alien" (21).

However, these worrying or defensive attitudes coexisted with much more hopeful responses. Indeed, as suggested in writings about the "hope-in-hopelessness" of people who face extinction (Crapanzano 2004, 111) or who have been cut off from leading religiously and morally worthwhile lives (Naumescu 2013), the spark of hope appears especially bright in "hopeless" situations. Moreover, it is in such destabilized contexts that hope has transformative potential by reorienting people to new horizons. In a way, the collapse of the state in Kyrgyzstan also "freed" people from their attachment to the state and the nation, and pushed them to redirect their hopes to new points of reference. As was illustrated throughout this book, the promises of health and wealth made by Pentecostal Christianity, the futures of affluence laid out by development workers, and the route to fulfillment suggested by Tablighi teachings proved to be very attractive to marginalized inhabitants.

These redirections of hope entailed more than mere projection. Engagement with new utopian points of reference was a productive process in which vague hope gained concreteness and agency. As Jarrett Zigon (2009, 256) has pointed out, rather than seeing hope as either passive or active, it is important to see how these aspects feed into and give way to each other over time.[9] People's engagement with religious and secular ideological movements allowed them to act on their hopes, "rendering hope—now recontextualized—into efficacious desire" as Crapanzano (2004, 120) formulates it. Hope was concretized through acts of praying and healing, by joining protests against the president, indeed, even by writing up a business plan for a United Nations development project. This is what Miyazaki (2004) refers to as the "method of hope," a process by which people attach themselves to this world and actively orient themselves toward the future.

The productive tensions between hope, desire, and reality were more than evident in the stories shared by Tablighi Muslims during their proselytizing trips (*dawats*), which focused on the inexplicable workings of the world, on frightening political events, and on relationships with women. To take the example of stories about sexual and caring relationships with women, these triggered the imagination precisely because such (idealized) relationships were wanting in the men's own lives. By sharing such stories within an all-male companionship and connecting them to the teachings of the Prophet, the desires became even more intense and tangible while remaining just out of reach, thereby keeping the tension alive. The tension remains productive as long as the object of desire remains unfulfilled yet within reach.

This last point is crucial because while the discrepancy between the ideal and the real keeps people motivated, the optimal distance between desire and its fulfillment is rarely maintained for a long period of time. Certainly, as we have seen, spiritual practitioners, Pentecostal preachers, Tablighi scholars, and development specialists worked hard to account for treatments that didn't cure and prayers that remained unanswered, and to explain why foreign investments did not materialize or why unexpected violence did occur. But such attempts could not always prevent the gap between desire and its realization from widening, potentially even become seen as unbridgeable. To understand these issues better, it is essential to explore how collective ideas reverberate within groups of like-minded people and are related to the temporal and spatial dynamics of ideological movements.

Reverberating: Effervescence and Its Aftermath

> It is certain my Conviction gains infinitely the moment another soul will believe in it.
>
> NOVALIS (1772–1801), QUOTED IN JOSEPH CONRAD, *LORD JIM* (1900)

Susan Buck-Morss has argued that "to define the enemy is, simultaneously, to define the collective. Indeed, defining the enemy is the act that brings the collective into being" (2000, 9). Analogously, challenges to the integrity of ideas can be powerful stimulants in the production of shared conviction. This logic surfaced in the discussion of the Tablighis, for whom challenges in the form of police detention and negative public preconceptions added to a sense of heroism, of belonging to a group of chosen people. Especially when congregating during their three-day mission trips, the collective facing of a hostile external world was exhilarating. Arguably, though, the logic of this principle was best phrased by Pastor Kadyrjan when he shared with me his thoughts on the matter: "We pray for [local government] officials to stop hindering us. But this may not be God's way. Our faith thrives when it is being repressed." It suggests, very concretely, that it is difference as such that keeps these movements alive, even in cases where difference takes the form of repression.[10]

The fervor produced through confrontation was also detected in the more long-term fluctuations of ideological movements. "Scientific atheism" reached its maximum momentum at times when its religious adversaries were, or were seen as, posing a real threat to modern society. As an ideological project, "scientific atheism" turned into a hollow shell once the battle against religion seemed to have been won. To retain some legitimacy, antireligious activists focused on "extreme forms" of religiosity, those that could continue to be seen as credibly dangerous adversaries. It is because of this that, ironically, atheism regained some of its attractions after it had been discarded. When the threat of excessive religiosity rose, some people realized that, after all, "what the communists taught us was right."

It will be useful to step back to reflect on how these points about difference relate to the arguments presented in the previous two sections, to then see how to move forward. The "voicing of hope" on the frontier was about the conceptualization and projection of new and different possibilities—a utopian horizon—and its hopeful and invigorating dimensions. Subsequently, the theme of difference was elaborated by discussing how tensions within constellations of ideas, as well as between these ideas and the prevalent social reality, contributed to collective ideas gaining traction. Moreover, these frictions or "encounters across difference" gained particular momentum when they were challenged, hence the role attributed to defining or being defined as an enemy.

What happens, concretely, is that in such instances the outward-oriented experience of difference recoils, thereby intensifying the inward-oriented experience of recognition or sameness.[11] Becoming aware of this mutuality, recognizing one's experiences in others, has an exhilarating effect. Let me repeat the epigraph of Conrad's *Lord Jim*, "It is certain my Conviction gains infinitely the moment another soul will believe in it."[12] This line is revealing because it emphasizes the *moment* of becoming aware of this mutuality, which is simultaneously a moment of distinction from all those others who do not share in the belief. Here, the push of distinction and the pull of sameness join forces to produce the effervescent quality of shared conviction.[13]

In this book, I have presented an ethnographic commentary on these points, demonstrating that the clarity and intensity of conviction is a dynamic and deeply social process. Using Weber's insights on charisma

(1968), I showed how the disruption of stable structures of rational-legal and traditional authority in Kyrgyzstan paved the way not only for charismatic authority but for "divinely given" experiences more generally. As in Bakhtin, it was with the falling away, or the suspension, of ordinary power structures that the "utopian ideal and the realistic merged," paving the way for festivals of the real ([1965] 1984). With Victor Turner I illustrated how in such situations the high and the low temporarily merge, allowing for inspired fellowship, an "intense comradeship and egalitarianism," to emerge (1969, 95). Crucially, the affective potential was never *fully* realized, thus partially preserving a state of anticipation, a process energized by its own internal contradictions.

The sense of clarity and conviction has momentary highs, as during miracle occurrences in the Pentecostal Church that lighten up as an epiphany, to then sink back into ambiguity and insignificance. There are moments when specific messages resonate within the body, affecting a person deeply, such as when a spiritual healer repeats something that a grandmother had said in one's childhood, or when a neophyte is overwhelmed by the kindness of the "brothers" and "sisters" in a congregation, or when young men are about to set fire to the houses belonging to people they had "always known was something wrong with." These flashes have creative, transformative, and destructive potential: fellow Pentecostal congregants *did* become like relatives who help each other in battling everyday problems; in the two Kyrgyz revolutionary situations not only did everything seem possible but the despised leaders *were* in fact removed from power; when simmering anxieties became projected on the Uzbek minority, hundreds of people *were* killed and thousands of houses burned.

The classic accounts of "antistructure" have argued that the emotive intensities associated with effervescence, charisma, and *communitas* "can seldom be maintained for very long" and that it is their fate to undergo "a 'decline and fall' into structure and law" (Turner 1969, 132). To an extent this principle has been borne out by the examples presented in this book. When in a state of conviction, people say and do things that in hindsight they are often surprised by. "It was *me* who spoke these words," exclaimed a previously committed antireligious teacher in surprise about what she had later come to see as vulgar materialist distortions. And a man who was still sympathetic to, but no longer deeply involved with, the Tablighi Jamaat told me, "When you are inside everything seems clear, everything connects, but afterward, when you have gained distance, it turns out to be more complicated." He was referring to the need to pay more attention to his family, and to no longer single-mindedly follow the tenets of his faith.

However, the ethnographic examples also suggested that the trajectories of conviction show important variation. The instable fervor becomes differently embedded in legal, customary, and hierarchical structures. The Church of Jesus Christ integrated miracle occurrences into a generalized discourse within the congregation; the intense experiences of the Tablighis were supposed to be repeated in a regular and predictable pattern. To an extent this was a trade-off, a balancing act that risked tipping over into indifference and disinterest. Still, in the unstable environment of Kyrgyzstan, complete routinization (and naturalization) of ideas rarely happened, and thus ideological currents were able to retain their potency.

The ideological movements discussed in this book had their own techniques for dealing with the tempering effects of routinization.[14] Pastor Kadyrjan's approach was to remain on the offensive, adopting a forward-moving strategy in which constantly new battles were sought and a pioneer mentality was fostered. Generating a continuous supply of impulses (such as miracle occurrence), the church had grown rapidly and produced an environment of constant fervor, yet one that was always on the brink of collapse and led to disillusion among those who could not keep up. The Tabighi Jamaat displayed a similar frontier mentality, but its practice of *dawat* revealed a somewhat different approach to tackle the balancing act. As in their "dry-dock" parable that spoke of the need of ships to regularly leave the rough sea to be patched up in a safe haven, so did their practice of *dawat* insist that adherents to the movement regularly retreat into the company of a fellowship and be nourished with spiritual food, providing them with strength to weather the storms of ordinary life. Ideological work in each of these movements was thus characterized by a form of pulsation, which served to maintain a sense of chosen-ness and uniqueness, and to perpetuate ideological fervor.

Let me end with a few final reflections on the notion of pulsation. For living organisms pulsation is a precondition of life: the impulse provides a boost of energy, and it is the retreating of energy that triggers a new pulsation: the inhalation of oxygen, the intake of food, the pumping of blood, the contraction of muscles. While movements such as those of Tablighis and Pentecostals devised their own ways of generating new impulses, the contraction did not always have to be generated from within as it was also produced in the confrontation with an external adversary—a combination, so to speak, of the "beat and the pulse."

Conviction, on the one hand, involves reaching out to a transcendental value, while on the other it implies a claim of uniqueness. The transcendental project provides a direction and a goal, while the assertion of uniqueness keeps the involved on their toes. Conviction is about keeping the external threat at bay; it is also about the utopian horizon that can be approached but that more often than not remains out of reach. These aspects work, however, in contradictory ways. The promise of the utopian horizon energizes, but its inaccessibility also frustrates and exhausts. The external threat provokes and stimulates up to a point, but once it becomes overwhelming it crushes communal integrity. The important point here is that convictions are not simply present, but are produced in dialogue with challenges.

And this, then, brings us back to the fragility of conviction. The efficacy of ideology should never be taken for granted: it takes arduous work, operating in the right conditions, to establish affective links between ideological messages and subjects. Ironically, at the very moment when ideational power reaches its greatest intensity, the risk of dissipation and disintegration reaches its peak as well, thereby setting in motion new cycles of affective belief and doubt.

NOTES

Introduction

1. KelKel, which translates as "renaissance," is a youth movement modeled on the Ukrainian and Georgian youth protest movements (which were influential during the Orange and Rose revolutions) and established for the purpose of fostering political change.

2. As is common practice in anthropology, I have replaced the names of my interlocutors with pseudonyms, except when they spoke in an official capacity or had asked me to use their actual name. In choosing pseudonyms I have tried to be mindful of their social, regional, and ethnic connotations.

3. As the last of the post-Soviet "color revolutions," after Georgia's Rose Revolution in 2003 and Ukraine's Orange Revolution in 2004, Kyrgyzstan's Tulip Revolution has been much commented on. See Pelkmans 2005; Cummings 2010; and Radnitz 2010.

4. In this book I use the term "affect" to refer to the emotive charges or "intensities" that arise in the complex interplay between human interiority and the exterior world and in which visceral and reflective responses merge. This use of the term implies that I distance myself from the central ideas promoted by authors associated with the affective turn, especially the idea that affect would be "prediscursive," a position that focuses too narrowly on the materiality of the brain and ignores how emotive charges or "intensities" are socially, culturally, and cognitively mediated. See Martin 2013 for a particularly compelling critique of the assumptions underlying the affective turn.

5. I use the term "frontier town" to invoke the power asymmetries and ideas of superiority that are implied in the term, and that were part and parcel of Soviet development, not least in Central Asia.

6. For example, Appadurai argues that "Islamic fundamentalism, Christian fundamentalism, and many other local and regional forms of cultural fundamentalism may be seen as a part of an emerging repertoire of efforts to produce previously unrequired levels of certainty about social identity, values, survival, and dignity" (2006, 7).

7. A related issue, associated with Louis Althusser's top-down or centered theory of the "ideological state apparatus," is that if all aspects of society are seen as contributing to a single over-arching ideological system, coherence tends to be overstated, thereby making it difficult to account for change. In response to these issues various alternatives have been proposed. Pierre Bourdieu, for instance, uses the terms "symbolic power" and "doxa" (unquestioned truth) to refer to the subtle and implicit ways by which ideational domination operates. Michel Foucault, rejecting Althusser's top-down and state-centered understanding of ideological power, adopts the more fluid and agentless concept of "discourse."

8. This was a central theme in post-Soviet literature. As Günther writes, "Emptiness may be considered to be a characteristic trait of the atmosphere of the 1990s when Russians felt to live in a cultural vacuum somewhere between state economy and unbridled capitalism" (2013: 100).

9. In the early 2010s others have written about the "rebirth of the Idea" as in a revival of ideological alternatives to the "corrupt, lifeless versions of 'democracy'" (Badiou 2012, 6).

10. This reflects Antonio Gramsci's notion of hegemony, which connects the direct (institutional) and indirect (cultural) ways by which the interests of the elite become part and parcel of the ideas of the people.

11. As Wolf suggests, "societies under increasing stress" caused by social, political, or ecological crisis often develop ideologies that are an extreme expression of underlying trends and tensions (1999, 274).

12. In the Marxist tradition ideology is traditionally seen as serving relations of domination, but as Eagleton argues, the ideas promoted by nondominant groups need not be less ideological, and he therefore defines ideology as being about "any kind of intersection between belief systems and political power" ([1991] 2007, 8).

13. It has been observed by others that interpellation works indeed almost effortlessly when these "types" or elements evoke each other and the chain of signification thus achieves "temporary coherence" (Finlayson 1996, 94; see also Laclau 1977, 102).

14. Althusser fails to convincingly explain why individuals would "accept as evident" the voice of ideology (Pêcheux 1994), with his theory presupposing "a prior and unelaborated doctrine of conscience" that is predicated on guilt (Butler 1995, 8). This unelaborated doctrine is reflected in his choice of examples—Christian sin and violation of the law—both of which suggest that the subject is drawn to ideology by being promised an identity that will soften this sense of guilt. But there is no reason why guilt should be singled out as the primary or even only emotive driver of "interpellation."

15. The term "utopian horizon" is inspired by Ernst Bloch's suggestion that "concrete utopia stands on the horizon of every reality" (1995, 223), as part of his emphasis on the role of the "Not-Yet" in history. As this suggests, I use "utopian" in a nonderogatory way to refer to imaginations and conceptualizations of a desired and better way of being (cf. Levitas 2011, 209).

16. The next day a new friend, from the train, made inquiries with the authorities. On learning that our undocumented traveling would get us into serious trouble, we decided to keep a low profile, staying in Kyrgyzstan for four weeks, before traveling back to Moscow by train.

1. Shattered Transition

1. This is not to say that all was quiet. The previous year (1990) had seen significant political unrest following ethnic conflict in Osh Province, with demonstrations demanding resignation of the first secretary Absamat Masaliev (Anderson 1999, 20; McGlinchey 2011, 77–78). But,

significantly, over 90% of the population voted in favor of retention of the Soviet Union (Cummings 2012, 52).

2. See www.youtube.com/watch?v=NEewvq_8CxU, accessed December 6, 2014. See also the newspapers *Delo No* August 27, 2003, 3 and *Vechernii Bishkek* August 14, 2003, 1–2.

3. Given that Bishkek had several prominently placed Manas statues already, erecting the hero on the central square in 2011 was not a novel statement, but it was a significant one given the central location and sensitive moment.

4. Morozova writes that the untimely rotation of monuments suggests "a failed attempt by the state at collective national identity construction" (2008, 18).

5. Alan Cranston and Michael Green, "Kyrgyzstan Takes Quiet Path to Democracy," *Christian Science Monitor*, May 4, 1994, http://www.csmonitor.com/1994/0504/04141.html.

6. Mikhail Gorbachev had frequently used the motto "The USSR is our common home" to express the view that in the Soviet Union the nationality question had been resolved (Zisserman-Brodsky 2003, 11).

7. Taken from an interview with Akaev by R. Sagdeev, June 24, 1997, that originally appeared on www.eisenhowerinstitute.org; also quoted in McBrien and Pelkmans 2008, 91.

8. This amounted to a decrease from 11,803,000 to 6,715,000 heads of cattle. The 63% decrease in sheep and goats was particularly steep. For an account of the impact on the village level, see Boris Petric's *Where Are All Our Sheep?* (2015).

9. Frederick Lamy suggests that local actors "mobilized into informal networks faster than state institutions were able to re-establish formal social and economic relations with communities," a process that "reinforced patterns of informality in state-society relations" (2013, 151).

10. McGlinchey (2011) argues that even the position of those who benefited most from privatization (such as the government) remained fragile. Although the government used economic resources to temporarily satisfy the elite, such rewards were insufficient to turn them into long-term loyal dependents.

11. Hirsch shows that by the early 1930s "even rural and nomadic populations that previously had not exhibited national consciousness were describing themselves as members of nationalities" (2005, 145).

12. This was not unlike the situation in post-Soviet Turkmenistan, about which Adrienne Edgar wrote that genealogy and tribal differences continued to be significant aspects of political ordering and were seen as a threat to national unity (2004, 264–65).

13. The term "European" is used locally to refer to Russians, Ukrainians, Germans, and people from the Baltic republics, in contrast to Turks, Caucasians, and Asians such as Kyrgyz, Uzbeks, and Kazakhs.

14. Estimates of the death toll from fighting in Osh, Jalalabad, and Bazar-Korgon in 2010 ranged from the official figure of 393 to one thousand (International Crisis Group 2010, 1, 18).

15. *Times of Central Asia*, April 4, 2005.

16. For in-depth analyses of the 2005 Tulip Revolution, see Radnitz 2010; Cummings 2010; and Pelkmans 2005. On the second Kyrgyz revolution, see Tabyshalieva 2013 and Reeves 2014b. On the 2010 conflict, see Gullette and Heathershaw 2015; McBrien 2011; and Abashin and Savin 2012.

17. International Crisis Group (2010) documented that most eyewitnesses agreed the conflict started as a fight between young Kyrgyz and Uzbek men in a gambling hall. When each side phoned their friends for assistance, the brawl started to escalate.

18. Daniel Kimmage, "Kyrgyzstan: The Failure of Managed Democracy," RFE/RL (Radio Free Europe / Radio Liberty), April 12, 2005, http://www.rferl.org, accessed June 10, 2005.

19. By 2009 my disillusioned acquaintances in the south were making jokes about the Bakiev family's greed, saying that Kyrgyzstan is too small a country for a president with seven (greedy) brothers.

2. Condition of Uncertainty

1. Emigration peaked in 1994, when, in the span of just nine months, Kokjangak's population dropped from 19,100 to 15,857 (Howell 1996, 63).

2. See also the works of Joshua Barker (2009, 47) and Janet Roitman (2006, 255), as these make similar claims about the structures of disorder in, respectively, Indonesia and Chad.

3. *Vechernii Bishkek*, July 6, 2001.

4. *Vechernii Bishkek*, October 16, 1997.

5. These lines of thought are further inspired by the work of Morten Pedersen (2012), Hirokazu Miyazaki (2004), and Henrik Vigh (2006), who each emphasize the reflective work that is triggered by personal and societal crises, and how this process activates aspirations, hopes, and desires.

6. In the late 1920s, when pressured to hand over his cattle to the newly established collective farm, Osman decided to chase his horses to an uninhabited mountain valley, hoping that things would have changed by the next spring. Things did not change, and most of his horses died during the cold winter.

7. *Kirgizskaia SSR* (Gos. izdatel'stvo geograficheskoi literatury, 1956).

8. For this purpose the town administration organized *voskresniki*, or "voluntary labor Sundays" (which coexisted with *subbotniki*, or "voluntary labor Saturdays"), ostensibly because of the enthusiasm of committed citizens, but surely also because labor was in short supply.

9. In 2004 approximately 160 men were involved in informal mining activities, but during the high season (in the fall) these numbers would go up. Arrangements varied from semi-professional brigades made up of former miners, to more informal groups of young men, called "apaches." The problems they faced were similar in that they mostly worked manually, without contracts, and without guarantees.

10. According to data compiled by the town administration (*otdel statistiki*), as of January 1, 2004, Kokjangak had 10,727 inhabitants, of which 75% (8,091) was classified Kyrgyz; 7% (804) Russian; 6% (670) Uzbek; 3% (347) Tatars; 2% (251) Kurds; 2% (198) Kazaks; 2% (159) Ukrainians; and some 200 people representing other nationalities.

11. This is consistent with other parts of Kyrgyzstan. Between 1989 and 1999 the official number of 688,000 people, the majority of which was Russian, emigrated (Schmidt and Sagynbekova 2008, 116).

12. Three of the four schools used Kyrgyz and one used Russian as the language of instruction, an inversion of the situation in Soviet times.

13. There had indeed been no open violence between Kyrgyz and Uzbeks in Kokjangak or other small industrial towns in 2010, despite the conflict having spread across both urban and rural settings across the region.

14. The joke was hardly funny but referred to the fact that most fifth-floor flats were occupied by single women (with or without children) and suggested that men ascending to this floor were visiting their (secret) lovers or in search of (paid) sex.

15. Apartments had been handed to their registered inhabitants in the early 1990s; industrial and communal buildings often remained public property. Many of these public buildings were "deregistered" in the 2000s, after which the construction materials were sold, with the profits usually ending up in the pockets of administrators.

16. Labor migration to Russia has become endemic throughout Kyrgyzstan, with an estimated one-third of the employable population working abroad, mostly in Russia (Schmidt and Sagynbekova 2008).

17. My use of the term "navigation" in this section is indebted to Vigh's stimulating discussion of social navigation in *Navigating Terrains of War* (2006), which is equally concerned with the relation between uncertainty and agency.

18. In most cases, the miners paid around 30% of their income to "officials" (*chinovniki*), which in this context means well-connected people who obtained the property rights of land that previously belonged to the state and had been managed through the "state forest" (*leskhoz*) administration.

19. In August 2007 the mayor closed the informal mining pits for a week after three men died, probably because news had reached the provincial government and news agencies, thus making (symbolic) action necessary. The effect of such temporary closures was that casualties were dealt with in confidence. For explicit reference to Kokjangak, however, see "Illegal Coal Mining Takes Several Lives but . . . ," which appeared several years earlier in the *Bishkek Observer*, April 5, 2004.

20. Hobbes refers to this saying in his work *De Cive* (1642/1651), which is also where he first mentions his idea of "war of all against all" (*bellum omnium contra omnes*).

21. As in Achille Mbembe's characterization of the postcolonial "chaotic plurality," there was an internal coherence, yet one that resulted not from a single specific order but was instead produced through the friction between different orders that were nevertheless inescapably linked (2006, 381). J.P. Olivier de Sardan's (1999) depiction of the postcolonial condition as "schizophrenic," that is, as a disempowering confrontation between an imposed (colonial) politico-legal structure and the locally prevalent sociocultural logics, also hints at the same problem.

22. Kokjangak was included in the program because of its reputation as one of the most destitute settlements in the region. Beyond this basic fact the UNDP workers knew little about the town and had no idea what to expect.

23. *Vechernii Bishkek*, October 16, 1997.

3. What Happened to Soviet Atheism?

1. Judging from the book's final paragraph, the manuscript must have gone to press shortly after October 9, 1990, when *Pravda* published the new law "about freedom of consciousness and religious organization." Melis Abdyldaev mentions that although this law may change the relationship with some facets of atheism, it was decided to publish the manuscript in its then-existing form (1991, 127).

2. Similar observations about the contradictory and counterproductive effects of antireligious propaganda have been made by Kendzior (2006) and Exnerova (2006, 106).

3. The trend is not restricted to the former Soviet Union. Western scholars used to be interested in the "what" and "how" of Soviet atheist ideology and antireligious policies, but the production of knowledge on these topics came to an abrupt end with the collapse of the USSR. While for Western religious scholars the failure of atheism was to be celebrated rather than questioned, for liberal atheists Soviet atheism was an embarrassment of sorts, because of its associations with totalitarianism. As if to illustrate this descent into oblivion, *The Cambridge Companion to Atheism* (Martin 2007a) does not even mention the Soviet experience.

4. One of Yurchak's telling examples concerns an interviewee who, while attending the Komsomol (Communist Youth League) meetings, hardly paid attention to what was being said, yet whenever a sign of affirmation was required, "a certain sensor would click in the head" telling him how to act (2003, 492).

5. See Yurchak's (2005, 102–18) discussion of the concept *svoi*, which he suggests is best translated as "those who belong to our circle," referring to a sense of intimacy and understanding among members.

6. Yurchak does not use the term "routinization" as such, but the idea is implied when he talks about the "progressively form-centered normalization of language" (2003, 490) in which ideological discourse became "hyper-normalized" (491).

7. It could be argued, with some justification, that this is a rather literal reading of Althusser that fails to sufficiently take into consideration his emphasis on the structural and material

underpinnings of ideology. However, the point of the literal reading is to make the concept of interpellation amenable to fragmented ideological landscapes, and to less than hegemonic assertions of ideology (as discussed in the introduction).

8. Similar distinctions have been suggested by others. Michael Martin (2007b) differentiates between positive and negative atheism, with negative atheism referring to a lack or absence of "theism," and positive atheism indicating an ideological stance, which can either be antireligious or substantively "atheist."

9. In contrast to my interviews with Olga Nikolaevna and Asel' Kosobaeva, this one was recorded in Bishkek, and is included in this chapter because it contains important complementary views.

10. The sacralization of secular leaders is, of course, not restricted to the Soviet Union. For example, Yael Navaro-Yashin writes about Ataturk that this "secular founder of [the Turkish] state was not remembered in a secularist fashion" (2002, 191).

11. Malte Rolf similarly shows that in the 1920s and 1930s the organizers of Soviet festivals made great efforts to compete with the buoyant religious-festival culture—an invigorating struggle, but with limited success (2000).

12. Although admiring the revolutionary power of Luther's reformation, Marx retained his ambivalence, as reflected in his statement that "if Protestantism was not the true solution it was at least the true setting of the problem" (Marx [1844] 1975, 182).

4. Walking the Truth in Islam with the Tablighi Jamaat

1. In contrast to the other chapters in this book, most of the research for this one was conducted outside of Kokjangak. The reason for this is that although Tablighis were active in Kokjangak, for my entrance to the group I depended on contacts in Bishkek. The three tours I participated in all took place in Chui Province, in northern Kyrgyzstan.

2. Dungans are a Chinese-speaking Muslim people. Most Dungans live in China, but several hundred thousand live in the Central Asian republics, including fifty thousand in Kyrgyzstan. Most of these Kyrgyz Dungans know Chinese, and all are fluent in Russian.

3. This Kyrgyz "joking relationship" with Islamic knowledge is reflected in the title of Maria Louw's 2012 text "Being Muslim the Ironic Way."

4. See Kirsch 2004 for a useful critique of static perspectives of belief.

5. The method of Tabligh, as its founder Mawlana Ilyas envisioned it in 1920s India, was explicitly designed to combat complacency and instill vigor, qualities that were seen to be lacking in other techniques such as education and *dhikr* (remembrance) (Masud 2000b, 7).

6. This is one reason why academic literature on the Tablighis is sparser than the size and influence of the movement would predict, as also Janson (2008) and Noor (2010) have observed.

7. The number ten thousand was mentioned by Igor Rotar (2007). Kadyr Malikov, director of the Center for Religion, Law, and Politics in Kyrgyzstan, gave me an estimate of fifteen thousand adherents in 2011.

8. According to Shamsibek Zakirov, an official with the State Agency for Religious Affairs, most Tablighis in Kyrgyzstan are ethnic Kyrgyz (Rotar 2007).

9. The corresponding view holds that the Kyrgyz would be less receptive to intense forms of religiosity than Uzbeks and Tajiks. The reason for this would be their nomadic past, a view that was popularized in Soviet times but also expounded by, for example, President Akaev. (See also chapter 1.)

10. The reported answer of the *dawatchi* was that the purpose of *dawat* is to learn rather than to teach others.

11. Emil Nasritdinov (2012) argues that an important reason for Tablighi success is their emphasis on traveling, as this resonates better with formerly nomadic people such as the Kyrgyz than with the traditionally stationary Uzbeks. However, since there are few actual pastoralists among

the Tablighis, it may be more accurate to speak of "nomadic nostalgia" (which is largely urban based) than actual nomadism.

12. This is not to deny that the movement can have an empowering effect for its female participants, as Mukaram Toktogulova (2014) demonstrates. The potential emancipatory effect is also stressed by scholars working in other regions, such as Marloes Janson, who reports (2008) that in the Gambia, *dawat* encourages gender emancipation because it transgresses boundaries between male and female tasks.

13. For an in-depth discussion of the changing configurations of "religion" and "culture" in Kyrgyzstan, see Khalid 2006, 84–115; and Pelkmans 2007.

14. The muftiate issued a recommendation to wear a Kyrgyz-style robe and a *kalpak*, instead of Pakistani dress, which was being discussed within Tablighi circles during my last visit, in 2013. Farish Noor comments (2010, 720) on similar tensions in Southeast Asia, which resulted in the Tablighis opting for local modes of dress.

15. Despite their "relentless apoliticism," which contributed to their harmless image (Metcalf 1996, 117), the Tablighis are seen by Kyrgyz authorities as potentially dangerous (Murzakhalilov and Arynov 2010). See Sikand 2003, for a discussion of this issue from a South Asian perspective.

16. The data presented in this section are largely based on one *dawat* in the summer of 2009, but have been augmented by two other three-day *dawats* I participated in, in 2009 and 2010.

17. The Tablighi jamaat has a clearly defined hierarchical structure in which at each level an *amir* takes charge, but this hierarchy is "mostly loose and temporary" (Masud 2000b, 28), with the *amir* expected to consider all opinions.

18. The *mashvara*, or council, is a central organizing feature of the Tablighis. Most decisions (at all levels) are made after consulting those involved, though the final decision rests with the *amir*.

19. The *baian*, or sermon, given by one person selected from the *jamaat*, discusses worldly life in relation to the hereafter, and is expected to highlight "the positive and negative aspects of the two worlds" (Masud 2000b, 27).

20. The six tenets are *kalmah*, article of faith; *salah*, the five daily prayers; *ilm* and *zikr*, knowledge and remembrance of Allah; *ikraam-e-Muslim*, respect for fellow Muslims; *Ikhlas-e-Niyyat*, or self-transformation; and *dawah* or *dawat*.

21. The food is particularly basic on the first day. Thereafter villagers tend to provide food, the quantity of which depends on local attitudes to *dawat*.

22. Barbara Metcalf usefully suggests that the interview has limited value in studies of the Tablighi Jamaat because researcher and respondents adhere to different speech conventions. Similar to what I experienced, her questions were often brushed aside as irrelevant (1996, 117–19).

23. Jacques Cousteau (1910–1997) was a French scientist and filmmaker who became famous in Europe and the former Soviet Union through his documentaries of maritime expeditions that were shown on television for many decades.

24. Similarly, Justine Quijada has argued that as a result of the Soviet atheist experience, "science and religion exist in a long-standing dialogic" and co-constitutive relationship to one another (2012, 148).

25. In 1990 at least six hundred people died in Uzgen and Osh. In 2010 at least 393 and up to one thousand people were killed in Osh, Jalalabad, and Bazar-Korgon (ICG 2010, 1, 18).

26. Such logic is mirrored in this suggestion made by *alim* Muhammad: "Muslims always win! If he wins in war, then he has the spoils of victory, while if he dies, he goes to heaven. A beggar is only happy if he is a Muslim. A president is only happy if he is a Muslim."

27. To quote Mohamed Tozy's rendering of the parable: "Man is a ship in trouble in tumultuous sea. It is impossible to repair it without taking it away from the high seas where the waves of ignorance and the temptations of temporal life assail it. Its only chance is to come back to land to be dry-docked. The dry-dock is the mosque of the jamaat" (Tozy 2000, 166).

28. I am indebted to Sondra Hausner for directing me to this line of analysis.

5. Pentecostal Miracle Truth on the Frontier

1. The official name is Full Gospel Church of Jesus Christ, but was commonly referred to as *Tserkov' Iisusa Khrista* (Church of Jesus Christ).

2. Or to quote Weber's phrasing, at times of distress the "natural" leaders "have been holders of specific gifts of the body and spirit" (1948, 245).

3. What I have in mind is the combination of assumed "superiority," self-ascribed creativity, and imagined independence that tends to characterize the missionary, colonial settler, and development worker. I rely here on work that draws, critically, on Frederick Jackson Turner's (1893) Frontier Thesis.

4. For example, church members mentioned being taken aback by the exuberant worshiping, and especially by "the speaking in tongues." Reflecting more widely held sentiments, one young male congregant mentioned that "the word 'God' was fine with me. But when Jesus's name was mentioned I would be scared. I feared that I was becoming a *kaffir* [infidel]."

5. As Robert Orsi has written, prayer is not an innocent psychological activity. Rather, "it is in and through prayer that the self comes into intimate and extended contact with the contradictions and constraints of the social world" (Orsi 1996, 186).

6. The development of such stable connections can refer to institutionalization in the Weberian sense, meaning that miracle occurrence gains bureaucratic authority by becoming embedded in church structures. It can also refer to a deepening of personal relationships with the divine. A good example is Tanya Luhrmann's analysis of "new paradigm" Christians in California who described "spiritual maturity" as having developed a long-term friendship with God in which "the problem of unanswered prayer becomes the problem of why your good buddy appears to be letting you down" (2007, 95).

7. This is not to say that there are no other ways to deal with disappointment. Naomi Haynes discusses the problem of disappointment with the prosperity gospel among Pentecostal Christians on the Zambian Copperbelt, showing how they adjusted their expectations to local economic and social realities, producing what she calls a "limited prosperity gospel" (2012, 127). Such adjustment of expectations also happened in the Church of Jesus Christ, but the differences between Jalalabad and Kokjangak show the limitations of such adjustment and hence the fragility of the church in destitute contexts.

8. The remaining 30% tended to have family members who converted before them, belong to Russian or Tatar minorities, or had kept their conversion secret from their relatives.

6. The Tenacity of Spiritual Healing and Seeing

1. I should mention that while Nurgul knew that I was "writing about religion," she was not fully aware of my financial situation and may have thought that my position was similar to those of the two Peace Corps Volunteers who were living in Kokjangak at the time.

2. In fact, Dinara had been painfully wrong a second time, when she saw that I did not have any children yet. When learning that I had two daughters, Sophie and Emma, living in a nearby town, she cleverly replied that I better take a DNA test.

3. In fact, most of my contacts with spiritual practitioners were established through acquaintances.

4. Elements of uncertainty and skepticism in post-Soviet "spirituality" have been noted by others. Marjorie Balzer writes that the Sakha she studies wonder about spiritual powers: "Are they real?" (2002, 144).

5. Similarly, Danuta Penkala-Gawęcka writes that in southern Kazakhstan "shamans were and still are highly esteemed" (2014, 42).

6. Zarcone (2013, xxv) mentions that the term *emchi* originates in Mongolia and means "healer," but is also commonly used in Tibet.

7. This flexibility of categories due to the borrowing from multiple sources has been noted by several others including Penkala-Gawęcka 2014, 38 and Biard 2013, 88.

8. In their discussion of shamanism in, respectively, Siberia and Mongolia, King (1999) and Pedersen (2011) observed a similar tendency among their informants to lament that there were no "real" shamans left. In the Mongolian case this created serious existential and ontological problems because "far too many spirits were on the loose [and] far too little shamanic knowledge and skill were available to rein in this occult excess" (Pedersen 2011, 8).

9. This energizing quality of doubt has been brilliantly illustrated by Giulia Liberatore in her discussion of pondering pious Somali Muslim women in London (2013).

10. However, other clairvoyants in the neighborhood were of the opinion that one of these orphans was *karmicheskii*—i.e., had a bad karma—and that this was affecting Marzia's powers negatively.

11. Stories about "shamanic sickness" are in fact very widespread, and constitute one of the elements through which the authenticity of a healer is assessed. See also Biard 2013.

12. These items are usually left by clients in the healer's house for a designated period of time in order to absorb powers that can then be used to fight off bad spirits.

13. I rely here on Chinara's memory because the whispered phrases were partly inaudible to me. In her appeals to invisible forces Marzia was assisted by the spirits of two holy women who showed her the way.

14. Perhaps I should mention that on the day of Akaev's arrival, the president's schedule was changed so that Chinara did not get a chance to actually give the talk.

15. A quantitative study of medical help–seeking behavior found that 25% of respondents in Kyrgyzstan mentioned financial difficulties as the main reason for their nonuse of biomedical services. An equal percentage mentioned not filling prescriptions because they were too expensive. The same study found that people in Tajikistan who made use of medical services spent as much money on informal payments as on formal payments for doctors and medicine combined (Falkingham 2002, 50–52).

16. For example, Vuillemenot (2013, 70–71) documents the story of a female *bakhsi* Khaiat living in southern Kazakhstan who had become temporarily deaf and ill as a teenager, was treated by two *bakhsis*, and recovered fully after accepting the role of *bakhsi*. She was unable to marry as a consequence.

17. It is in light of similar observations that Patrick Garrone writes: "In the fight for the supremacy over souls, Islam gains advantages from its more institutional nature, its financial power, its capacity to penetrate the highest levels of society and the international support it enjoys" (2013, 18). Although I observed similar differences, in my analysis the absence of institutionalization is ironically also the strength of "shamanism."

Conclusion

1. The term "frontier" is useful precisely because it is politically suspect, refracting reality through the prism of asserted superiority and (assumed) dominance. When this is kept in mind, the term highlights that we are talking about encounters playing out in a tilted and unstable zone of asymmetric forces. See Chappell (1993, 270) and Baud and Van Schendel (1997, 213) for elements of this definition of the frontier, and its critical grounding in Frederick Jackson Turner's (1921) discussion of the frontier in US history.

2. Kadyrjan told me that he could always tell if someone was from Kokjangak by shaking hands: the hands of people from Kokjangak were noticeably colder than those of people living elsewhere—a clear sign of the presence of evil.

3. Risbek (Richard Hewitt) wrote several books about this, the first of which appeared in English and in Kyrgyz as *Ak Kalpak* in 2003. He subsequently wrote a more elaborate account,

Manas Lost and Found: A Bridge Linking Kyrgyzstan's Epic to Ancient Oracles, which was also self-published, and appeared in 2012. For a short discussion of "Manas-Christianity," see Pelkmans 2007.

4. Three years after this encounter one of these *dawatchis* told me that such a spiritual awakening was under way in Ak-Tiuz: a new mosque had been constructed (with money from an external source), which was said to be increasingly used for the Friday prayers by the town's inhabitants.

5. On "resource frontiers," Anna Tsing insightfully writes that frontiers "create wildness so that some—and not others—may reap its rewards" (2005, 27).

6. This idea has long been acknowledged in the study of borders, where it is argued that the existence of borders as barriers to movement simultaneously creates the reasons for crossing them (Donnan and Wilson 1999, 87).

7. Wittgenstein's observations about the need for friction in order to make progress in logical investigations are suggestive here: "We have got onto slippery ice where there is no friction and so in a certain sense the conditions are ideal, but also, just because of that, we are unable to walk. We want to walk so we need friction. Back to the rough ground!" (Wittgenstein [1953] 2010, 46).

8. It is quite evident that a similar balancing played a role in what made the Pentecostal Church attractive. Some of its practices, such as speaking in tongues, were confounding to novices, while its message of empowerment was closely tuned to popular ideas of spiritual realities.

9. While agreeing with Zigon that the passive and active dimensions of hope should be seen in relation to hope's temporal aspects (2009, 256), I disagree with him that Crapanzano (2004) fails to address this. In fact Crapanzano shows persuasively how undefined and silent hope may gain in concreteness and agency. It is just that when Crapanzano discusses these complex processes he uses the English term "desire" for the more concrete forms of the "not-yet," while Zigon prefers to continue with the term "hope."

10. This "being defined as the enemy" is the corollary to Buck-Morss's suggestion (2000, 9) that "to define the enemy" brings the collective into being.

11. These findings point to what Laclau refers to as the constitutive role played by social heterogeneity in the construction of "the 'people'" (2005, 223). For him collective identity gains in intensity when facing an "antagonistic frontier" as this provides direction to collective action (80, 84–85).

12. I am grateful to Jim Lance for bringing this quotation to my attention. Appropriately, the line has been associated as much with Joseph Conrad, the doubter who uses it as the epigraph of his book *Lord Jim*, as with its writer, Novalis, the man with a mission who wrote the line as a thought fragment.

13. The reader might have expected more engagement with Durkheim's collective effervescence, not least because of his emphasis on reverberation: "each re-echoes the others, and is re-echoed by the others. The initial impulse thus proceeds, growing as it goes, as an avalanche grows in its advance" (1915, 215–16). However, Durkheim assumes that the "emotional and passional faculties of the primitive" allow for effervescence to simply arise in the act of congregation (215), an obviously problematic view that is unhelpful in understanding the strengths and weaknesses of collective ideas.

14. In Weber's sociology, "routinization" refers to the process by which charisma becomes embedded in or absorbed by rational-legal and traditional structures. Weber argues that the charismatic does not completely evaporate but can be enhanced by these other registers of authority (1968, 54–61).

REFERENCES

Abashin, S.N., and I.S. Savin. 2012. "Osh, 2010: Konfliktuiushchaia etnichnost'." In *Etnichnost' i religiia v sovremennykh konfliktakh*, edited by V.A. Tishkov and V.A. Shnirel'man, 23–56. Moscow: Nauka.

Abdyldaev, Melis. 1991. *Iz istorii religii i ateizma v Kyrgyzstane*. Bishkek: Ilim.

Abrams, Philip. 1988. "Notes on the Difficulty of Studying the State." *Journal of Historical Sociology* 1 (1): 58–89.

Adams, Laura. 2010. *The Spectacular State: Culture and National Identity in Uzbekistan*. Durham, NC: Duke University Press.

Akaev, Askar. 1993. "Kyrgyzstan: Central Asia's Democratic Alternative." *Democratizatsiya: The Journal of Post-Soviet Democratization* 1 (Winter 1993): 9–23.

———. 1995. *Kyrgyzstan: Na puti stanovleniya nezavisimosti: Izbrannye vystupleniya i rechi Prezidenta Kyrgyzskoi Respubliki Askara Akaeva*. Bishkek: Uchkun.

———. 2003. *Kyrgyzskaia Gosudarstvennost' i Narodnyi Epos "Manas."* Bishkek: Uchkun.

Alexander, Catherine. 2009. "Waste under Socialism and After: A Case Study from Almaty." In *Enduring Socialism: Explorations of Revolution and Transformation, Restoration and Continuation*, edited by Harry West and P. Raman, 148–68. New York: Berghahn Books.

Ali, Jan. 2011. "Piety among Tablighi Women." *Contemporary Islam* 5:225–47.

Althusser, Louis. (1971) 2008. "Ideology and Ideological State Apparatuses (Notes towards an Investigation)." In *On Ideology*, 1–60. London: Verso.

Anderson, Benedict. (1983) 2006. *Imagined Communities: Reflections on the Origin and Spread of Nationalism*. London: Verso.

Anderson, John. 1999. *Kyrgyzstan: Central Asia's Island of Democracy?* Amsterdam: Harwood Academic Publishers.

Appadurai, Arjun. 2006. *Fear of Small Numbers: An Essay on the Geography of Anger*. Durham, NC: Duke University Press.

Badiou, Alain. 2012. *The Rebirth of History: Times of Riots and Uprisings*. London: Verso.

Baggini, Julian. 2009. *Atheism: A Brief Insight*. New York: Sterling Publishing.

Bakhtin, Mikhail Mikhaĭlovich. (1968) 1984. *Rabelais and His World*. Translated by Hélène Iswolsky. Bloomington: Indiana University Press.

Balci, Bayram. 2012. "La jama'at al Tabligh en Asie centrale: Réactivation des liens islamiques avec le sous continent indien et insertion dans un islam mondialisé." *Revue des mondes musulmans et de la Méditerranée* 130:181–99.

Balzer, Marjorie Mandelstam. 2002. "Healing Failed Faith? Contemporary Siberian Shamanism." *Anthropology and Humanism* 26 (2): 134–49.

Barker, Joshua. 2009. "Negara Beling: Street-Level Authority in an Indonesian Slum." In *State of Authority: The State in Society in Indonesia*, edited by Gerrie van Klinken and Joshua Barker, 47–72. Southeast Asia Program Publications. Ithaca, NY: Cornell University Press.

Baud, Michiel, and Willem Van Schendel. 1997. "Toward a Comparative History of Borderlands." *Journal of World History* 8 (2): 211–42.

Bell, Daniel. 1960. *The End of Ideology: On the Exhaustion of Political Ideas in the Fifties*. Cambridge, MA: Harvard University Press.

Bercken, William van den. 1985. "Ideology and Atheism in the Soviet Union." *Religion, State and Society* 13 (3): 269–81.

Biard, Aurelie. 2013. "Interrelation to the Invisible in Kirghizistan." In *Shamanism and Islam: Sufism, Healing Rituals and Spirits in the Muslim World*, edited by T. Zarcone and A. Hobart, 79–94. London: IB Tauris.

Bloch, Alexia. 2005. "Longing for the Kollektiv: Gender, Power, and Residential Schools in Central Siberia." *Cultural Anthropology* 20 (4): 534–69.

Bloch, Ernst. 1995. *The Principle of Hope*. Volume 1. Translated by Neville Plaice, Stephen Plaice, and Paul Knight. Cambridge, MA: MIT Press.

Bloch, Maurice. 2008. "Why Religion Is Nothing Special but Is Central." *Philosophical Transactions of the Royal Society B: Biological Sciences* 363 (1499): 2055–61.

———. 2013. *In and Out of Each Other's Bodies: Theory of Mind, Evolution, Truth, and the Nature of the Social*. Boulder, CO: Paradigm.

Borenstein, Eliot. 1999. "Suspending Disbelief: 'Cults' and Postmodernism in Post-Soviet Russia." In *Consuming Russia: Popular Culture, Sex and Society since Gorbachev*, edited by A. Barker, 437–62. Durham, NC: Duke University Press.

Bourdieu, Pierre. 1977. *Outline of a Theory of Practice*. Cambridge: Cambridge University Press.

Boyer, Pascal. 1994. *The Naturalness of Religious Ideas: A Cognitive Theory of Religion*. Berkeley: University of California Press.

Boym, Svetlana. 2001. *The Future of Nostalgia*. New York: Basic Books.

Brubaker, Rogers. 2004. *Ethnicity without Groups*. Cambridge, MA: Harvard University Press.

———. 2011. "Nationalizing States Revisited: Projects and Processes of Nationalization in Post-Soviet States." *Ethnic and Racial Studies* 34 (11): 1785–1814.

Buchli, Victor. 2007. "Astana: Materiality and the City." In *Urban Life in Post-Soviet Asia*, edited by C. Alexander, V. Buchli, and C. Humphrey, 40–69. London: Routledge.

Buckley, Mary, ed. 1997. *Post-Soviet Women: From the Baltic to Central Asia*. Cambridge: Cambridge University Press.

Buck-Morss, Susan. 2000. *Dreamworld and Catastrophe: The Passing of Mass Utopia in East and West*. Cambridge, MA: MIT Press.

Burawoy, Michael, and Pavel Krotov. 1992. "The Soviet Transition from Socialism to Capitalism: Worker Control and Economic Bargaining in the Wood Industry." *American Sociological Review* 57 (1): 16–38.

Butler, Judith. 1995. "Conscience Doth Make Subjects of Us All." *Yale French Studies* 88:6–26.

Carothers, Thomas. 2002. "The End of the Transition Paradigm." *Journal of Democracy* 13 (1): 5–21.

Chappell, David. 1993. "Ethnogenesis and Frontiers." *Journal of World History* 4 (2): 267–75.

Chormonov, B.S., and A.F. Sidorov. 1963. *Promyshlennyi Progress v Kirgizskoi SSR*. Frunze: Kirgizskoe Gosudarsvennoe Izdatel'stvo.

Chotaeva, Cholpon. 2004. *Ethnicity, Language and Religion in Kyrgyzstan*. Sendai, Japan: Tohoku University.

Coleman, Simon. 2003. "Continuous Conversion? The Rhetoric, Practice, and Rhetorical Practice of Charismatic Protestant Conversion." In *The Anthropology of Religious Conversion*, edited by A. Buckser and S. Glazier, 15–27. Lanham, MD: Rowman and Littlefield.

Comaroff, Jean, and John L. Comaroff. 2000. "Millennial Capitalism: First Thoughts on a Second Coming." *Public Culture* 12 (2): 291–343.

Connery, Joyce. 2000. "Caught between a Dictatorship and a Democracy: Civil Society, Religion and Development in Kyrgyzstan." *Praxis: The Fletcher Journal of Human Security* 16:1–18.

Cooley, Alexander, and James Ron. 2002. "The NGO Scramble: Organizational Insecurity and the Political Economy of Transnational Action." *International Security* 27 (1): 5–39.

Crapanzano, Vincent. 2004. *Imaginative Horizons: An Essay in Literary-Philosophical Anthropology*. Chicago: University of Chicago Press.

Csordas, Thomas J. 2007. "Introduction Modalities of Transnational Transcendence." *Anthropological Theory* 7 (3): 259–72.

Cummings, Sally, ed. 2010. *Domestic and International Perspectives on Kyrgyzstan's "Tulip Revolution."* London: Routledge.

———. 2012. *Understanding Central Asia: Politics and Contested Transformations*. London: Routledge.

———. 2013. "Leaving Lenin: Elites, Official Ideology and Monuments in the Kyrgyz Republic." *Nationalities Papers* 41 (4): 606–21.

Davie, Grace. 2012. "Belief and Unbelief: Two Sides of a Coin." *Approaching Religion* 2 (1): 3–7.

Donham, Donald. 1999. *Marxist Modern: An Ethnographic History of the Ethiopian Revolution*. Berkeley: University of California Press.

Donnan, Hastings, and Thomas Wilson. 1999. *Borders: Frontiers of Identity, Nation and State*. Oxford: Berg.

Douglas, Mary. 1966. *Purity and Danger: An Analysis of Concepts of Pollution and Taboo*. London: Routledge.

———. 1975. *Implicit Meanings: Selected Essays in Anthropology*. London: Routledge.

Duffin, Jacalyn. 2007. "The Doctor Was Surprised; Or, How to Diagnose a Miracle." *Bulletin of the History of Medicine* 81 (4): 699–729.

Durkheim, Emile. 1915. *The Elementary Forms of the Religious Life*. London: George Ellen & Unwin.

Eagleton, Terry. (1991) 2007. *Ideology: An Introduction*. New and updated edition. London: Verso.

Edgar, Adrienne. 2004. *Tribal Nation: The Making of Soviet Turkmenistan*. Princeton, NJ: Princeton University Press.

Eisenstadt, S.N. 1968. Introduction. In *Max Weber: On Charisma and Institution Building*, edited by S.N. Eistenstadt, ix–lvi. Chicago: University of Chicago Press.

Engelke, Matthew. 2014. "Christianity and the Anthropology of Secular Humanism." *Current Anthropology* 55 (S10): S292–S301.

Ewing, Katherine. 1994. "Dreams from a Sufi Saint: Anthropological Atheism and the Temptation to Believe." *American Anthropologist* 96 (3): 571–84.

Exnerova, Vera. 2006. "Caught between the Muslim Community and the State: The Role of Local Uzbek Authorities in Ferghana Valley, 1950s–1980s." *Journal of Muslim Minority Affairs* 26 (1): 101–12.

Falkingham, Jane. 2002. "Poverty, Affordability and Access to Health Care." In *Health Care in Central Asia*, edited by M. McKee, J. Healy, and J. Falkingham, 42–56. Buckingham, England: Open University Press.

Farrington, John D. 2005. "De-development in Eastern Kyrgyzstan and Persistence of Semi-nomadic Livestock Herding." *Nomadic Peoples* 9 (1–2): 171–97.

Ferguson, James. 1990. *The Anti-Politics Machine: "Development," Depoliticization, and Bureaucratic Power in Lesotho*. Cambridge: Cambridge University Press.

———. 2004. "Transnational Topographies of Power: Beyond 'the State' and 'Civil Society' in the Study of African Politics." In *A Companion to the Anthropology of Politics*, edited by J. Vincent, 383–99. Malden, MA: Blackwell.

Finlayson, Alan. 1996. "Nationalism as Ideological Interpellation: The Case of Ulster Loyalism." *Ethnic and Racial Studies* 19 (1): 88–112.

Fitzpatrick, Sheila. 1999. *Everyday Stalinism: Ordinary Life in Extraordinary Times; Soviet Russia in the 1930s*. New York: Oxford University Press.

Foucault, Michel. 1978. *The History of Sexuality*. Vol. 1, *An Introduction*. Translated by Robert Hurley. New York: Vintage.

Fukuyama, Francis. 1989. "The End of History?" *National Interest* 16:1–18.

Gaborieau, Marc. 2000. "The Transformation of Tablighi Jama'at into a Transnational Movement." In *Travellers in Faith: Studies of the Tablighi Jama'at as a Transnational Islamic Movement for Faith Renewal*, edited by Muhammad Khalid Masud, 121–38. Leiden: Brill.

Garrone, Patrick. 2013. "Healing in Central Asia: Syncretism and Acculturation." In *Shamanism and Islam: Sufism, Healing Rituals and Spirits in the Muslim World*, edited by T. Zarcone and A. Hobart, 17–46. London: IB Tauris.

Geertz, Clifford. 1973. *The Interpretation of Cultures*. New York: Basic Books.

Gellner, Ernest. 1983. *Nations and Nationalism*. Ithaca, NY: Cornell University Press.

Grant, Bruce. 1995. *In the Soviet House of Culture: A Century of Perestroikas*. Princeton, NJ: Princeton University Press.

———. 2001. "New Moscow Monuments, or, States of Innocence." *American Ethnologist* 28 (2): 332–62.

———. 2010. "Cosmopolitan Baku." *Ethnos* 75 (2): 123–47.

Gregg, Melissa, and Gregory Seigworth. 2010. "An Inventory of Shimmers." *The Affect Theory Reader*, edited by Melissa Gregg and Gregory Seigworth, 1–25. Durham, NC: Duke University Press.

Gullette, David. 2010. *The Genealogical Construction of the Kyrgyz Republic: Kinship, State and "Tribalism."* Folkestone, England: Global Oriental.

Gullette, David, and John Heathershaw. 2015. "The Affective Politics of Sovereignty: Reflecting on the 2010 Conflict in Kyrgyzstan." *Nationalities Papers* 43 (1): 122–39.

Günther, Hans. 2013. "Post-Soviet Emptiness (Vladimir Makanin and Viktor Pelevin)." *Journal of Eurasian Studies* 4 (1): 100–106.

Hage, Ghassan. 2003. *Against Paranoid Nationalism: Searching for Hope in a Shrinking Society*. Pluto Press.

Hann, Chris, and Mathijs Pelkmans. 2009. "Realigning Religion and Power in Central Asia: Islam, Nation-State and (Post) Socialism." *Europe-Asia Studies* 61 (9): 1517–41.

Harding, Susan. 1987. "Convicted by the Holy Spirit: The Rhetoric of Fundamental Baptist Conversion." *American Ethnologist* 14 (1): 167–81.

Hastrup, Kirsten. 2004. "Getting It Right: Knowledge and Evidence in Anthropology." *Anthropological Theory* 4 (4): 455–72.

Haynes, Naomi. 2012. "Pentecostalism and the Morality of Money: Prosperity, Inequality, and Religious Sociality on the Zambian Copperbelt." *Journal of the Royal Anthropological Institute* 18:123–39.

Heide, Nienke van der. 2008. "Spirited Performance: The Manas Epic and Society in Kyrgyzstan." PhD thesis, University of Amsterdam.

Heyat, Farideh. 2004. "Re-Islamisation in Kyrgyzstan: Gender, New Poverty and the Moral Dimension." *Central Asian Survey* 23 (3–4): 275–87.

Hirsch, Francine. 1997. "The Soviet Union as a Work-in-Progress: Ethnographers and the Category Nationality in the 1926, 1937, and 1939 Censuses." *Slavic Review* 56 (2): 251–78.

———. 2005. *Empire of Nations: Ethnographic Knowledge and the Making of the Soviet Union*. Ithaca, NY: Cornell University Press.

Hirschkind, Charles. 2011. "Media, Mediation, Religion." *Social Anthropology* 19 (1): 90–97.

Hobbes, Thomas. 1651. *Leviathan; or, The Matter, Forme and Power of a Common Wealth Ecclesiasticall and Civill.* London: printed for Andrew Crooke, at the Green Dragon in St.Pauls Church-yard. Prepared for the McMaster University Archive of the History of Economic Thought, by Rod Hay.

Howell, Jude. 1996. "Poverty and Transition in Kyrgyzstan: How Some Households Cope." *Central Asian Survey* 15 (1): 59–73.

Humphrey, Caroline. 1991. "'Icebergs,' Barter, and the Mafia in Provincial Russia." *Anthropology Today* 7 (2): 8–13.

———. 1998. *Marx Went Away—But Karl Stayed Behind.* Ann Arbor: University of Michigan Press.

———. 1999. "Shamans in the City." *Anthropology Today* 15 (3): 3–10.

———. 2002. *The Unmaking of Soviet Life: Everyday Economies after Socialism.* Ithaca, NY: Cornell University Press.

Husband, William. 2000. *"Godless Communists": Atheism and Society in Soviet Russia, 1917–1932.* DeKalb: Northern Illinois University Press.

International Crisis Group (ICG). 2010. "The Pogroms in Kyrgyzstan." *Asia Report* 193 (August 23). http://www.crisisgroup.org/~/media/Files/asia/central-asia/kyrgyzstan/193%20The%20Pogroms%20in%20Kyrgyzstan.ashx.

Ismailbekova, Aksana. Forthcoming. *Blood Ties and the Native Son: Poetics of Patronage in Kyrgyzstan.* Bloomington: Indiana University Press.

Janson, Marloes. 2006. "The Prophet's Path: Tablighi Jamaat in the Gambia." *ISIM Review* 17:44–45.

———. 2008. "Renegotiating Gender: Changing Moral Practice in the Tablighi Jamaat in the Gambia." *Journal for Islamic Studies* 28:9–36.

Jost, John. 2006. "The End of the End of Ideology." *American Psychologist* 61 (7): 651–70.

Kalb, Don. 2005. "From Flows to Violence: Politics and Knowledge in the Debates on Globalization and Empire." *Anthropological Theory* 5 (2): 176–204.

Kamp, Marianne. 2006. *The New Woman in Uzbekistan: Islam, Modernity, and Unveiling under Communism.* Seattle: University of Washington Press.

Kapferer, Bruce. 1988. *Legends of People, Myths of State: Violence, Intolerance, and Political Culture in Sri Lanka and Australia.* New York: Berghahn Books.

———. 2003. "Introduction: Outside All Reason—Magic, Sorcery and Epistemology in Anthropology." In *Beyond Rationalism: Rethinking Magic, Witchcraft and Sorcery*, edited by Bruce Kapferer, 1–30. New York: Berghahn Books.

Karagiannis, Emmanuel. 2009. *Political Islam in Central Asia: The Challenge of Hizb Ut-Tahrir.* London: Routledge.

Karpat, Kemal. 1993. "The Old and New Central Asia." *Central Asian Survey* 12 (4): 415–25.

Kashirin, F.T. 1988. "Ugol'naya geologiya v Kirgizii za 70 let Sovetskoy vlasti." *Izvestiya Akademii nauk Kirgizskoy SSR* 1:72–79.

Kendzior, Sarah. 2006. "Redefining Religion: Uzbek Atheist Propaganda in Gorbachev-Era Uzbekistan." *Nationalities Papers* 34 (5): 533–48.

Khalid, Adeeb. 2006. *Islam after Communism: Religion and Politics in Central Asia.* Berkeley: University of California Press.

King, Alexander. 1999. "Soul Suckers: Vampiric Shamans in Northern Kamchatka, Russia." *Anthropology of Consciousness* 10 (4): 57–68.

Kirsch, Thomas. 2004. "Restaging the Will to Believe: Religious Pluralism, Anti-Syncretism, and the Problem of Belief." *American Anthropologist* 106 (4): 699–709.

Kocaoglu, Timur. 1984. "Islam in the Soviet Union: Atheistic Propaganda and 'Unofficial' Religious Activities." *Journal of Muslim Minority Affairs* 5 (1): 145–52.

Kosmarskaia, Natal'ia. 2006. *"Deti imperii" v postsovetskoi Tsentral'noi Azii: Adaptivnye praktiki i mental'nye sdvigi: Russkie v Kirgizii, 1992–2002)*. Moscow: Natalis Press.

Kotkin, S. 1995. *Magnetic Mountain: Stalinism as Civilization*. Berkeley: University of California Press.

Kristof, Ladis K.D. 1959. "The Nature of Frontiers and Boundaries." *Annals of the Association of American Geographers* 49:269–82.

Kyrgyzstan Inquiry Commission. 2011. "Report of the Independent International Commission of Inquiry into Events in Southern Kyrgyzstan in June 2010." http://reliefweb.int/report/kyrgyzstan/report-independent-international-commission-inquiry-events-southern-kyrgyzstan.

Laclau, Ernesto. 1977. *Politics and Ideology in Marxist Theory: Capitalism, Fascism, Populism*. London: New Left Books.

———. 1993. "Politics and the Limits of Modernity." In *Postmodernism: A Reader*, edited by T. Docherty. New York: Columbia University Press.

———. 2005. *On Populist Reason*. London: Verso.

Lamy, Frederick. 2013. "Social Networking Practices: Continuity or Rupture with the Soviet Past?" In *Social and Cultural Change in Central Asia: The Soviet Legacy*, edited by S. Akyildiz and R. Carlson, 145–59. London: Routledge.

Lane, Christel. 1981. *The Rites of Rulers: Ritual in Industrial Society—the Soviet Case*. Cambridge: Cambridge University Press.

Laszczkowski, Mateusz. 2011. "Building the Future: Construction, Temporality, and Politics in Astana." *Focaal: Journal of Global and Historical Anthropology* 60:77–92.

Lawrence, John. 1972. "Observations on Religion and Atheism in Soviet Society." *Canadian Slavonic Papers/Revue Canadienne des Slavistes* 14 (4): 577–85.

Ledeneva, Alena. 1998. *Russia's Economy of Favours: Blat, Networking and Informal Exchange*. Cambridge: Cambridge University Press.

———. 2006. *How Russia Really Works: The Informal Practices That Shaped Post-Soviet Politics and Business*. Ithaca, NY: Cornell University Press.

Levitas, Ruth. 2011. *The Concept of Utopia*. Oxford: Peter Lang.

Lewis, David. 2008. *The Temptations of Tyranny in Central Asia*. New York: Columbia University Press.

Liberatore, Giulia. 2013. "Doubt as a Double-Edged Sword: Unanswerable Questions and Practical Solutions among Newly Practising Somali Women in London." In *Ethnographies of Doubt: Faith and Uncertainty in Contemporary Societies*, edited by M. Pelkmans, 225–50. London: IB Tauris.

Lindquist, Galina. 2001. "The Culture of Charisma: Wielding Legitimacy in Contemporary Russian Healing." *Anthropology Today* 18 (2): 3–8.

——. 2006. *Conjuring Hope: Healing and Magic in Contemporary Russia*. New York: Berghahn Books.

Liu, Morgan. 2012. *Under Solomon's Throne: Uzbek Visions of Renewal in Osh*. Pittsburgh: University of Pittsburgh Press.

Louw, Maria. 2010. "Dreaming Up Futures: Dream Omens and Magic in Bishkek." *History and Anthropology* 21 (3): 277–92.

——. 2012. "Being Muslim the Ironic Way: Secularism, Religion and Irony in Post-Soviet Kyrgyzstan." *Varieties of Secularism in Asia: Anthropological Explorations of Religion, Politics and the Spiritual*, edited by Nils Bubandt and Martijn van Beek, 143–61. London: Routledge.

Luehrmann, Sonja. 2011. *Secularism Soviet Style: Teaching Atheism and Religion in a Volga Republic*. Bloomington: Indiana University Press.

Luhrmann, Tanya. 2007. "How Do You Learn to Know That It Is God Who Speaks?" In *Learning Religion: Anthropological Approaches*, edited by D. Berliner and R. Sarró, 83–102. New York: Berghahn Books.

Marat, Erica. 2008. "Imagined Past, Uncertain Future: The Creation of National Ideologies in Kyrgyzstan and Tajikistan." *Problems of Post-Communism* 55 (1): 12–24.

Marsden, Magnus. 2008. "Muslim Cosmopolitans? Transnational Life in Northern Pakistan." *Journal of Asian Studies* 67 (1): 213–47.

Martin, Emily. 2013. "The Potentiality of Ethnography and the Limits of Affect Theory." *Current Anthropology* 54 (S7): S149–S158.

Martin, Michael, ed. 2007a. *The Cambridge Companion to Atheism*. Cambridge: Cambridge University Press.

——. 2007b. "Atheism and Religion." In *The Cambridge Companion to Atheism*, edited by M. Martin, 217–32. Cambridge: Cambridge University Press.

Martin, Terry. 2001. *The Affirmative Action Empire: Nations and Nationalism in the Soviet Union, 1923–1939*. Ithaca, NY: Cornell University Press.

Marx, Karl. (1844) 1975. "Contribution to the Critique of Hegel's Philosophy of Law: Introduction." In *Marx and Engels Collected Works*, 175–87. Moscow: Progress Publishers.

——. (1844) 2002. "Critique of Hegel's Philosophy of Right." In *Marx on Religion*, edited by John Raines, 170–82. Philadelphia: Temple University Press.

Masud, Muhammad Khalid. 2000a. Introduction. In *Travellers in Faith: Studies of the Tablighi Jama'at as a Transnational Islamic Movement for Faith Renewal*, edited by M. Masud, xiii–lx. Leiden: Brill.

——. 2000b. "The Growth and Development of the Tablighi Jama'at in India." In *Travellers in Faith: Studies of the Tablighi Jama'at as a Transnational Islamic Movement for Faith Renewal*, edited by M. Masud, 3–43. Leiden: Brill.

Matveeva, Anna. 2010. "Kyrgyzstan in Crisis: Permanent Revolution and the Curse of Nationalism." Working paper 79. Crisis States Working Papers Series 2. LSE Destin.

Mbembe, Achille. 2006. "The Banality of Power and the Aesthetics of Vulgarity in the Postcolony." In *The Anthropology of the State: A Reader*, edited by A. Sharma and A. Gupta, 381–400. Malden, MA: Blackwell.

McBrien, Julie. 2006. "Listening to the Wedding Speaker: Discussing Religion and Culture in Southern Kyrgyzstan." *Central Asian Survey* 25 (3): 341–57.

———. 2011. "Leaving for Work, Leaving in Fear." *Anthropology Today* 27 (4): 3–4.

———. 2013. "Afterword: In the Aftermath of Doubt." In *Ethnographies of Doubt: Faith and Uncertainty in Contemporary Societies*, edited by M. Pelkmans, 251–68. London: IB Tauris.

McBrien, Julie, and Mathijs Pelkmans. 2008. "Turning Marx on His Head: Missionaries, 'Extremists,' and Archaic Secularists in Post-Soviet Kyrgyzstan." *Critique of Anthropology* 28 (1): 87–103.

McGlinchey, Eric. 2011. *Chaos, Violence, Dynasty: Politics and Islam in Central Asia*. Pittsburgh: University of Pittsburgh Press.

Metcalf, Barbara. 1993. "Living Hadith in the Tablighi Jama'at." *Journal of Asian Studies* 52 (3): 584–608.

———. 1996. "New Medinas: The Tablighi Jama'at in America and Europe." In *Making Muslim Space in North America and Europe*, edited by B. Metcalf, 110–30. Berkeley: University of California Press.

———. 2002. "'Traditionalist' Islamic Activism: Deoband, Tablighis, and Talibs." ISIM Papers 4. Institute for the Study of Islam in the Modern World.

Meyer, Birgit. 1998. "'Make a Complete Break with the Past': Memory and Post-Colonial Modernity in Ghanaian Pentecostalist Discourse." *Journal of Religion in Africa* 28 (3): 316–49.

Mitchell, Timothy. 1990. "Everyday Metaphors of Power." *Theory and Society* 19 (5): 545–77.

Miyazaki, Hirokazu. 2004. *The Method of Hope: Anthropology, Philosophy, and Fijian Knowledge*. Stanford, CA: Stanford University Press.

Moldobaev, I. 2002. "Religioznye verovaniia Kyrgyzov s drevneishikh vremen do segodniashnykh dnei." *Tsentral'naia Aziia i Kultura Mira* 1–2 (12–13): 137–43.

Morozova, Irina. 2008. "National Monuments and Social Construction in Mongolia and Kyrgyzstan." *IIAS Newsletter* 49:18–19.

Mosko, Mark. 2005. "Introduction: A (Re)Turn to Chaos: Chaos Theory, the Sciences, and Social Anthropological Theory." In *On the Order of Chaos: Social Anthropology and the Science of Chaos*, edited by M. Mosko and F. Damon, 1–46. New York: Berghahn Books.

Murzakhalilov, Kanatbek, and Mirajiddin Arynov. 2010. "Tablighi Jamaat in Kyrgyzstan: Its Local Specifics and Possible Impact on the Religious Situation." *Central Asia and the Caucasus* 11 (3): 162–67.

Murzakulova, Asel, and John Schoeberlein. 2009. "The Invention of Legitimacy: Struggles in Kyrgyzstan to Craft an Effective Nation-State Ideology." *Europe-Asia Studies* 61 (7): 1229–48.

Nasritdinov, Emil. 2012. "Spiritual Nomadism and Central Asian Tablighi Travelers." *Ab Imperio* 2012 (2): 145–67.

Naumescu, Vlad. 2013. "Old Believers' Passion Play: The Meaning of Doubt in an Orthodox Ritualist Movement." In *Ethnographies of Doubt: Faith and Uncertainty in Contemporary Societies*, edited by M. Pelkmans, 85–118. London: IB Tauris.

Navaro-Yashin, Yael. 2002. *Faces of the State: Secularism and Public Life in Turkey*. Princeton, NJ: Princeton University Press.

———. 2012. *The Make-Believe Space: Affective Geography in a Post-War Polity*. Durham, NC: Duke University Press.

Nazpary, Joma. 2002. *Post-Soviet Chaos: Violence and Dispossession in Kazakhstan*. London: Pluto Press.

Noor, Farish. 2010. "On the Permanent Hajj: The Tablighi Jama'at in South East Asia." *South East Asia Research* 18 (4): 707–34.

Olaveson, Tim. 2001. "Collective Effervescence and Communitas: Processual Models of Ritual and Society in Emile Durkheim and Victor Turner." *Dialectical Anthropology* 26 (2): 89–124.

Olivier de Sardan, J.P. 1999. "A Moral Economy of Corruption in Africa?" *Journal of Modern African Studies* 37 (1): 25–52.

Orsi, Robert. 1996. *Thank You, Saint Jude: Women's Devotion to the Patron Saint of Hopeless Causes*. New Haven, CT: Yale University Press.

Pêcheux, Michel. 1994. The Mechanism of Ideological (Mis)Recognition." In *Mapping Ideology*, edited by S. Žižek, 141–51. Verso.

Pedersen, Morten Axel. 2011. *Not Quite Shamans: Spirit Worlds and Political Lives in Northern Mongolia*. Ithaca, NY: Cornell University Press.

———. 2012. "A Day in the Cadillac: The Work of Hope in Urban Mongolia." *Social Analysis* 56 (2): 136–51.

Pelkmans, Mathijs. 2005. "On Transition and Revolution in Kyrgyzstan." *Focaal: Journal of Global and Historical Anthropology* 46:147–57.

———. 2006a. *Defending the Border: Identity, Religion, and Modernity in the Republic of Georgia*. Ithaca, NY: Cornell University Press.

———. 2006b. "Asymmetries on the 'Religious Market' in Kyrgyzstan." In *The Postsocialist Religious Question: Faith and Power in Central Asia and East-Central Europe*, edited by C. Hann, 29–46. Berlin: Lit Verlag.

———. 2007. " 'Culture' as a Tool and an Obstacle: Missionary Encounters in Post-Soviet Kyrgyzstan." *Journal of the Royal Anthropological Institute* 13 (4): 881–99.

———. 2009a. "Introduction: Post-Soviet Space and the Unexpected Turns of Religious Life." In *Conversion after Socialism: Disruptions, Modernisms, and the Technologies of Faith*, edited by M. Pelkmans, 1–16. New York: Berghahn Books.

———. 2009b. "Temporary Conversions: Encounters with Pentecostalism in Muslim Kyrgyzstan." In *Conversion after Socialism: Disruptions, Modernisms, and the Technologies of Faith*, edited by M. Pelkmans, 143–61. New York: Berghahn Books.

———. 2013. "Outline for an Ethnography of Doubt." In *Ethnographies of Doubt: Faith and Uncertainty in Contemporary Societies*, edited by M. Pelkmans, 1–42. London: IB Tauris.

Penkala-Gawęcka, Danuta. 2013. "Mentally Ill or Chosen by Spirits? 'Shamanic Illness' and the Revival of Kazakh Traditional Medicine in Post-Soviet Kazakhstan." *Central Asian Survey* 32 (1): 37–51.

———. 2014. "The Way of the Shaman and the Revival of Spiritual Healing in Post-Soviet Kazakhstan and Kyrgyzstan." *Shaman* 22 (1–2): 35–61.

Peris, Daniel. 1998. *Storming the Heavens: The Soviet League of the Militant Godless*. Ithaca, NY: Cornell University Press.

Petric, Boris. 2015. *Where Are All Our Sheep? Kyrgyzstan, a Global Political Arena*. New York: Berghahn Books.

Pomfret, Richard. 2006. *The Central Asian Economies since Independence*. Princeton, NJ: Princeton University Press.

———. 2007. "Central Asia since the Dissolution of the Soviet Union: Economic Reforms and Their Impact on State-Society Relations." *Perspectives on Global Development and Technology* 6 (1): 313–43.

Popov, Vladimir. 2000. "Shock Therapy versus Gradualism: The End of the Debate (Explaining the Magnitude of Transformational Recession)." *Comparative Economic Studies* 42 (1): 1–58.

Port, Mattijs van de. 1994. *Het Einde van de Wereld: Beschaving, redeloosheid en zigeuner-cafes in Servie*. Amsterdam: Babylon-De Geus.

———. 1998. *Gypsies, Wars, and Other Instances of the Wild: Civilization and Its Discontents in a Serbian Town*. Amsterdam: Amsterdam University Press.

Pospielovsky, Dimitry. 1987. *A History of Soviet Atheism in Theory and Practice, and the Believer*. Vol. 1, *A History of Marxist-Leninist Atheism and Soviet Anti-Religious Policies*. New York: St. Martin's Press.

Powell, David. 1967. "The Effectiveness of Soviet Anti-Religious Propaganda." *Public Opinion Quarterly* 31 (3): 366–80.

Quijada, Justine. 2012. "Soviet Science and Post-Soviet Faith: Etigelov's Imperishable Body." *American Ethnologist* 39 (1): 138–54.

Radnitz, Scott. 2010. *Weapons of the Wealthy: Predatory Regimes and Elite-Led Protests in Central Asia*. Ithaca, NY: Cornell University Press.

Rasanayagam, Johan. 2006. "Healing with Spirits and the Formation of Muslim Selfhood in Post-Soviet Uzbekistan." *Journal of the Royal Anthropological Institute* 12 (2): 377–93.

Reeves, Madeleine. 2008. "Border Work: An Ethnography of the State at Its Limits in the Ferghana Valley." PhD thesis, University of Cambridge.

———. 2014a. *Border Work: Spatial Lives of the State in Rural Central Asia*. Ithaca, NY: Cornell University Press.

———. 2014b. " 'We're with the people!' Place, Nation, and Political Community in Kyrgyzstan's 2010 'April Events.' " *Anthropology of East Europe Review* 32 (2): 68–88.

Robbins, Joel. 2007. "Continuity Thinking and the Problem of Christian Culture: Belief, Time, and the Anthropology of Christianity." *Current Anthropology* 48 (1): 5–38.

Ro'i, Yaacov. 1984. "The Task of Creating the New Soviet Man: 'Atheistic Propaganda' in the Soviet Muslim Areas." *Soviet Studies* 36 (1): 26–44.

Roitman, Janet. 2006. "The Ethics of Illegality in the Chad Basin." In *Law and Disorder in the Postcolony*, edited by Jean Comaroff and John Comaroff, 247–72. Chicago: University of Chicago Press.

Rolf, Malte. 2000. "Constructing a Soviet Time: Bolshevik Festivals and Their Rivals during the First Five-Year Plan; A Study of the Central Black Earth Region." *Kritika: Explorations in Russian and Eurasian History* 1 (3): 447–73.

Rotar, Igor. 2007. "Pakistani Islamic Missionary Group Establishes a Strong Presence in Central Asia." July 23. Eurasianet.org. http://www.eurasianet.org/departments/insight/articles/eav072307a.shtml.

Roy, Olivier. 2000. *The New Central Asia: Geopolitics and the Birth of Nations*. London: IB Tauris.

Schmidt, Matthias, and Lira Sagynbekova. 2008. "Migration Past and Present: Changing Patterns in Kyrgyzstan." *Central Asian Survey* 27 (2): 111–27.

Shahrani, Nazif. 1995. "Islam and the Political Culture of 'Scientific Atheism' in Post-Soviet Central Asia: Future Predicaments." In *The Politics of Religion in Russia and the New States of Eurasia*, edited by M. Bourdeaux, 273–92. Armonk, NY: M.E. Sharpe.

Shishkin, Philip. 2013. *Restless Valley: Revolution, Murder, and Intrigue in the Heart of Central Asia*. New Haven, CT: Yale University Press.

Sikand, Yoginder. 2003. "The Tablighi Jama'at and Politics." *ISIM Review* 13:42–43.

Slezkine, Yuri. 1994. "The USSR as a Communal Apartment; or, How a Socialist State Promoted Ethnic Particularism." *Slavic Review* 53 (2): 414–52.

Smith, Jesse M. 2013. "Creating a Godless Community: The Collective Identity Work of Contemporary American Atheists." *Journal for the Scientific Study of Religion* 52 (1): 80–99.

Somfai Kara, David. 2013. "Religious Traditions among the Kazakhs and the Kirghizs." In *Shamanism and Islam: Sufism, Healing Rituals and Spirits in the Muslim World*, edited by T. Zarcone and A. Hobart, 47–58. London: IB Tauris.

Spector, Regine. 2004. "The Transformation of Askar Akaev, President of Kyrgyzstan." *Berkeley Program in Soviet and Post-Soviet Studies Working Paper Series*. Berkeley: University of California.

Sperber, Dan. 1985. "Anthropology and Psychology: Towards an Epidemiology of Representations." *Man* (n.s.) 20:73–89.

Spoor, Max. 1995. "Agrarian Transition in Former Soviet Central Asia: A Comparative Study of Uzbekistan and Kyrgyzstan." *Journal of Peasant Studies* 23 (1): 46–63.

Tabyshalieva, Anara. 1993. *Vera v Turkestane: Ocherk istorii religii Srednei Azii i Kazakhstana*. Bishkek: Az-Mak.

———. 2013. "Kyrgyzstan between Revolutions." In *From Perestroika to Rainbow Revolutions: Reform and Revolution after Socialism*, edited by V. Cheterian, 143–73. London: Hurst.

Thompson, Karen, P. Schofield, N. Foster, and G. Bakieva. 2006. "Kyrgyzstan's Manas Epos Millennium Celebrations: Post-Colonial Resurgence of Turkic Culture and the Marketing of Cultural Tourism." In *Festivals, Tourism and Social Change: Remaking Worlds*, edited by D. Picard and M. Robinson, 172–90. Towbridge, England: Cromwell Press.

Toktogulova, Mukaram. 2014. "The Localisation of the Transnational Tablighi Jama'at in Kyrgyzstan: Structures, Concepts, Practices and Metaphors." In *Crossroads Asia Working Paper Series*, no. 17. Bonn.

Tozy, Mohamed. 2000. "Sequences of a Quest: Tablighi Jama'at in Morocco." In *Travellers in Faith: Studies of the Tablighi Jama'at as a Transnational Islamic Movement for Faith Renewal*, edited by M. Masud, 161–73. Leiden: Brill.

Tsing, Anna. 2005. *Friction: An Ethnography of Global Connection*. Princeton, NJ: Princeton University Press.

Turner, Edith. 2012. *Communitas: The Anthropology of Collective Joy*. London: Palgrave Macmillan.

Turner, Frederick Jackson. 1921. *The Frontier in American History*. New York: Henry Holt.

Turner, Victor. 1969. *The Ritual Process: Structure and Anti-Structure*. New Brunswick, NJ: Transaction Publishers.

Verdery, Katherine. 1996. *What Was Socialism and What Comes Next?* Princeton, NJ: Princeton University Press.

———. 1999. *The Political Lives of Dead Bodies: Reburial and Postsocialist Change*. New York: Columbia University Press.

Vigh, Henrik. 2006. *Navigating Terrains of War: Youth and Soldiering in Guinea-Bissau*. New York: Berghahn Books.

Vorontsova, Lyudmila, and Sergei Filatov. 1994. "Religiosity and Political Consciousness in Postsoviet Russia." *Religion, State and Society* 22 (4): 397–402.

Vries, Hent de. 2001. "In Media Res: Global Religion, Public Spheres, and the Task of Contemporary Religious Studies." In *Religion and Media*, edited by H. de Vries and S. Weber, 4–42. Stanford, CA: Stanford University Press.

Vuillemenot, Anne-Marie. 2013. "Muslim Shamans in Kazakhstan." In *Shamanism and Islam: Sufism, Healing Rituals and Spirits in the Muslim World*, edited by T. Zarcone and A. Hobart, 59–78. London: IB Tauris.

Wachtel, Andrew. 2013. "Kyrgyzstan between Democratization and Ethnic Intolerance." *Nationalities Papers* 41 (6): 971–86.

Wanner, Catherine. 2007. *Communities of the Converted: Ukrainians and Global Evangelism*. Ithaca, NY: Cornell University Press.

———. 2011. "Multiple Moralities, Multiple Secularisms." In *Multiple Moralities and Religions in Post-Soviet Russia*, edited by J. Zigon, 214–23. New York: Berghahn Books.

Weber, Max. 1948. *From Max Weber: Essays in Sociology*. Translated, edited, and with an introduction by H. Gerth and C. Wright Mills. London: Routledge and Kegan Paul.

———. 1968. *On Charisma and Institution Building*. Chicago: University of Chicago Press.

Wedel, Janine. 2001. *Collision and Collusion: The Strange Case of Western Aid to Eastern Europe*. London: Palgrave Macmillan.

Wikan, Unni. 1996. "The Nun's Story." *American Anthropologist* 98 (2): 279–89.

Willerslev, Rane. 2007. *Soul Hunters: Hunting, Animism and Personhood among the Siberian Yukaghirs*. Berkeley: University of California Press.

Wittgenstein, Ludwig. (1953) 2010. *Philosophical Investigations*. Hoboken, NJ: John Wiley & Sons.

Wolf, Eric. 1999. *Envisioning Power: Ideologies of Dominance and Crisis*. Berkeley: University of California Press.

Yanovskaya, Mariya. 2009. "'Tablighi Jamaat': Hidden Threat of Peaceful Preaching." February 16. *Ferghana News Agency*. http://enews.fergananews.com/articles/2505.

Yurchak, Alexei. 2003. "Soviet Hegemony of Form: Everything Was Forever, Until It Was No More." *Comparative Studies in Society and History* 45 (3): 480–510.

———. 2005. *Everything Was Forever, Until It Was No More: The Last Soviet Generation.* Princeton, NJ: Princeton University Press.

Zarcone, Thierry. 2013. Introduction. In *Shamanism and Islam: Sufism, Healing Rituals and Spirits in the Muslim World*, edited by T. Zarcone and A. Hobart, xxi–xxxi. London: IB Tauris.

Zigon, Jarrett. 2009. "Hope Dies Last: Two Aspects of Hope in Contemporary Moscow." *Anthropological Theory* 9 (3): 253–71.

Zisserman-Brodsky, Dina. 2003. *Constructing Ethnopolitics in the Soviet Union: Samizdat, Deprivation and the Rise of Ethnic Nationalism*. London: Palgrave Macmillan.

Žižek, Slavoj. 1994. "Introduction: The Spectre of Ideology." In *Mapping Ideology*, edited by S. Žižek, 1–33. London: Verso.

———. 2001. *On Belief*. London: Routledge.

INDEX

affect, 9, 70, 125; concept of, 185n4
affective dimension, 2–3, 5, 10, 37, 92
affective potential, 181
affective qualities, 5, 36, 91, 122, 171, 183
Akaev, Askar, 1–2, 19–26, 30, 34–39; on religion, 190n9
Akaev government, 20, 23–24, 42, 61, 141
Althusser, Louis, 7, 10–11, 84–85, 101, 186n7, 186n14, 189n7
atheism: "actually existing," 79, 81; disappearance of, 79–83; indifference to, 82, 83; Islam and, 115; object of ridicule, 77–79; scientific, 79–82, 86–88, 92, 96, 101, 180
atheist activists, 77, 80, 82

Bakiev, Kurmanbek, 1–4, 20, 35, 37, 39, 187n19
bakshi, 138, 151–56, 161–62, 166–67; meaning of, 151; "real," 154, 155. *See also* shaman
Bishkek: central square in, 17–21, 187n3; migration to, 67, 88, 138–39; mosques in, 105, 109–10, 117, 118; Pentecostal church in, 126, 130, 135
bribery, 66. *See also* corruption
bureaucracy: authority and, 162, 192n6; ideal-typical, 67; Soviet, 55, 65; structures of, 55, 67

capitalism, 29, 40–41, 186n8; empty signifier, 41–42; "late," 8; rhetoric of, 169; transition to, 26; victory of, 6
chaos, 4, 37, 60, 69, 174; inner, 114; order and, 65, 68; post-Soviet, 4, 47, 61, 65, 68, 130–31, 146
chaos theory, 68
charisma, 9–10, 123, 125, 128, 181; authority and, 125–26, 180–81, 194n14; divine gift, 125
charisma paradox, 140
church: buildings, 81, 89, 124, 126; "home," 130, 132, 134, 139; leadership, 126, 133–36, 140–41
civilization, 4, 86, 173; extraterrestrial, 89
civilized behavior, 36, 38, 41, 57, 175
civil service, 28
civil society, 13, 25
clairvoyants, 152–54, 158, 164–67; believability of, 151, 162, 164; pastor mistaken for, 136; relations amongst, 164, 169; visions of, 165, 166. *See also* spiritual practitioners
coal mining. *See* mining
collective effervescence. *See* effervescence
collective ideas: affective dimension of, 2–3, 170; attraction of, 12; intensity of, 2, 171, 179–80; people's connection with, 10; power and, 170; strength of, 171, 194n13